INTERMITTENT ~~FASTING~~ BLASTING

RECIPES

OPTIMIZE YOUR INTERMITTENT BLAST WITH OVER 100 DELICIOUS RECIPES: JUICES, SMOOTHIES, SOUPS AND MORE!

WILLIAM KING

Copyright © 2017 The Nutra Company, Inc. All rights reserved, including the right to reproduce this book or portions thereof in any form whatsoever.

This publication contains the opinions and ideas of its author and publisher. The information, products, and recipes contained and referenced in this publication are intended to be helpful and informative for anyone interested in the Intermittent Blasting. This book is sold with the understanding that the author and publisher are not engaged in dispensing health or medical advice or services. The information and advice contained in this book are intended as a general guide to Intermittent Blasting, dieting, and healthier eating and are not specific to individuals or their particular circumstances. This book is not intended to replace treatment by a qualified practitioner. If you know or suspect that you have a health problem, you should consult a health professional.

The author and publisher make no warrants or representations as to the completeness or accuracy of this book's contents, and specifically disclaim any and all warranties of any kind, expressed or implied. The information, recipes, references, and products contained in this book may not be suitable for every reader, as each individual reader's general health and condition will be unique to them. Each reader should consult his or her physician or health care practitioner before attempting Intermittent Blasting or any of the suggestions in this book or drawing inferences from them. The author and publisher specifically disclaim any liability, loss or risk, personal or otherwise, incurred as a consequence, directly or indirectly of the use and application of any of the contents of this book.

Visit us online at IntermittentBlasting.com

Acknowledgments

This book only exists due to the many contributions of David Iversen, Barbara Frey Waxman, PhD, Professor of English Emerita, University of North Carolina - Wilmington, Sally Beare and Amy Greene. Each contributed greatly with their unique talents and specialized expertise.

David's creativity was instrumental in organizing, editing, wordsmithing, formatting the book for print and designing the cover.

As an English Professor, Barbara was essential in finalizing the grammatical structure of this book.

With her extensive knowledge of nutrition through her work as a nutritional therapist, author and renowned expert on Longevity Hot Spots, Sally contributed nutritional content and also provided recipes.

Amy contributed several delicious recipes as well as helped with descriptions and organizing.

Table of Contents

Acknowledgments iii
Table of Contents v
Chapter 1: Introduction 1
    Welcome to Intermittent Blasting! Super Nutritious, Super Delicious Recipes 1
Chapter 2: Smoothies and Juicing 3
    Intermittent Blasting Smoothies 3
    Juicing 4
    Purchasing Fresh Cold-Pressed Juice 5
    How to Juice 5
    Great Juice Ingredients 6
    Juicing Tips 6
    Benefits of Commonly Used Fruits and Vegetables in Smoothies and Juice 7
        Apples 8
        Beets 8
        Carrots 8
        Celery 9
        Cucumber 9
        Lemons 9
        Kale 10
        Parsley 10
        Spinach 11
Chapter 3: Intermittent Blasting Recipes 13
    Smoothies 13
        Simple Smoothie 13
        Lemon Green 13
        Fruit and Salad Smoothie With Mint 14
        Strawberry Watermelon Smoothie 14
        Metal Detox 14
        Fresh Almond Milk with Veggies and Berries 14
        Green Tea Blast! 15
        Blueberry Piña Colada Blast 15
        Raw Anti-Inflammatory Recovery Drink 15
        Strawberry-Mango 16
        Cherry Pomegranate 16
    Quick and Easy Smoothies (4 Ingredients or Less) 16
        Delicious Kale Mango 16
        Mango Apple Blast 16
        Mango Coconut Blast 16
        Training Smoothie 17

Intermittent Blasting Recipes

Electrolyte Grape-Ginger Lemonade 17
Pineapple Blast 17
Green Juices **17**
   Newbie Green 18
   Simple Green 18
   Greens with Carrot 18
   Green Lemonade 18
   Greens with Pea Sprouts 19
   Green Detox 19
   Dr. Oz's Green Drink 19
   Greens and Berries 20
   Coconut Green 20
   Greens With A Kick 20
   Veggies and Greens 20
   Greens with Ginger 21
   Super Liver Support 21
   Beets and Greens 21
   Delicious Green Tea 21
Quick and Easy Juices (4 Ingredients or Less) **22**
   Greens and Grapefruit 22
   Fruit Peppermint 22
   Watermelon Cucumber with Mint 22
   Apple Strawberry 22
   Orange Pineapple Blast 23
   Liver Cleanse 23
   LemonAid 23
   Pineapple Mango 23
   Quick Apple Strawberry 24
   Quick Carrot Apple 24
   Beet Apple Blast! 24
   Quick Apple Pear 24
   Apple Carrot with Ginger 24
   Carrot Spinach with Kale 24
   Strawberry Watermelon Blast 24
   Carrots with Greens 24
   Cabbage, Celery, Lime 25
   Apple, Celery, Cucumber 25
   Romaine, Celery, Apple 25
   Celery, Carrot, Apple 25
   Pineapple Strawberry 25
   Carrot Cucumber Beet 25
   Carrot Beet Parsley 25

Intermittent Blasting Recipes

- Romaine, Cabbage, Carrot 26
- Carrot, Apple, Potato (yes, potato) 26

Dinner Juices **26**
- Healthy Veggie (V-8) 26
- V3 with Lemon 26
- V4 27
- Kale, Carrots, Celery 27
- Asparagus Juice 27
- Carrot, Celery, Romaine 27
- Carrot, Parsley, Romaine, Lemon 27
- Swiss Chard, Carrot, Celery 27
- Salsa Fresh 27
- Blast O' Veggies 28

Soups **28**
- Creamy Broccoli 28
- Tomato Basil 29
- Raw Creamy Cucumber Avocado 29
- Super Green 30
- Raw Almond Pea Soup 30
- Creamed Spinach Soup 30
- Watermelon Mango Soup 31
- Avocado Mint 31
- Raw Sweet Potato Soup 32
- Raw Green Veggie Soup 32

Chapter 4: After The Intermittent Blast **34**

Transitional Smoothies **34**
- Fruit Smoothie 101 34
- Banana Berry 34
- Coconut Milk Pina Colada 35
- Strawberry Coconut 35
- Blueberry Coconut Smoothie 35
- Fruit Salad with Mint 35
- Banana Lime Cinnamon 36
- Coconut Kale Blast! 36
- Delicious Chocolate Blast! 36
- Healthy Chocolate Banana Blast! 36
- Creamy Coconut Strawberry Blast! 37
- Banana Berry Fruit Smoothie 37
- Chocolate Almond Banana Blast 37
- The Banana Berry 37
- Cranberry-Green Tea 38
- Banana Peach 38

Intermittent Blasting Recipes

 Strawberry Banana 38
 Coconut Banana 38
 Blueberry Mango Blast 39
 Banana Cream Pie 39
 Blackberry-Mango 39
 Strawberry-Banana 39
 Vanilla Fruit 40
 Jump-Start your Day! 40
 Pineapple Kale 40
Hot-Spot Smoothie Recipes 40
 The Okinawa Tropical 40
 The Symi Minty Green 41
 The Campodimele Tomato and Herb 41
 The Sardinia Red Grape 41
 The Nicoya Avocado 41
 The Loma Linda Nut and Cinnamon 42
 The Hunza Apricot 42
 The Bama Exotic Fruit 42
Transitional Soups 42
 Bone Broth / Bone Marrow Soup 43
 Simple Veggie Soup 44
 Ratatouille 45
 Leek, Potato, and Watercress 45
 Zucchini Soup 46
 Tomato Soup 46
 Quick Bean and Tomato Soup 47
 Mung Bean Soup 48
 Gazpacho 49
 Roasted Beet Soup 49
 Sweet Potato and Carrot Soup 50
 Acorn Squash Soup 50
 Thai Sweet Potato and Carrot Soup 51
 Miso Soup with Noodles 52
Salads / Salad Dressings 52
 Simple Olive Oil and Lemon Dressing 53
 Olive Oil and Raw Apple-Cider Vinegar Dressing 53
 Avocado Sesame Salad 53
 Mediterranean Salad 54
 Greek Salad 54
 Tomato and Basil Salad 55
 Beet and Carrot Salad 55
 Baby Spinach, Watercress, and Arugula Salad 56

Intermittent Blasting Recipes

Fennel, Artichoke, and Lentil Salad 56
Zucchini and Carrot Salad 56
Japanese Salad 57
Cucumber and Wakame Salad 57
Bean Sprout Salad 58
Summer Peach and Tomato Salad 58
Greek Salad, Symi Style 58
Tuna Nicoise Salad 59
Quick Salad with Beans or Lentils 59

Transition Entrees 60
Lentil Shepherd's Pie 60
Salmon with Lentils 61
Adzuki Bean Burgers 62
Gallo Pinto (Costa Rican rice and beans) 63
Buckwheat Wraps 64
Amy's Lemon-Rosemary Salmon 64

Chapter 5: Healthy Eating Every Day! 66
Snacks 66
Guacamole 67
Salsa 68
Traditional Hummus 69
Dairy-Free Pesto 69
Chunky Sweet Potato Salsa 69
Dahl with Lemon and Coriander 70

Healthy Treats 71
No-Bake Fudge Brownies 71
Go Green Ice Pops 72
Strawberry Basil Ice Pops 72
Banana Oatmeal Raisin Cookies 73
Three-Berry Chia Pudding 73
No-Bake Cinnamon Apple Dessert 73

Chapter 6: Superfoods 75
The Amazing Power of Superfoods 75
What Exactly Are Superfoods? 75
Acai Berries 75
Apples 76
Apricots 76
Avocados 77
Blueberries 78
Beans 79
Brassica Vegetables 80
Buckwheat 81

Intermittent Blasting Recipes

Chocolate (cacao) 81
Chlorella and Spirulina 82
Cinnamon 84
Flax..84
Garlic...85
Ginger..87
Goji Berries..87
Green Tea..88
Mushrooms 89
Spinach..90
Sprouted Foods..91
Sweet Potatoes..92
Tomatoes and Tomato Paste 93
Turmeric..93
Fermented foods 94
Superfood References.. 95
Chapter 7: Healthy Life Overview.. 101
ABB - "Always Be Blasting"...101
Living a Healthy Life 101
A Healthy Diet in a Nutshell...101
Become a Locavore 106
Buy Organic When Possible 106
How to Prepare Vegetables 108
Oven-Roasted Vegetables...108
Stir-fried vegetables 108
Steamed vegetables 109
Beans and Lentils..109

Chapter 1: Introduction

Welcome to Intermittent Blasting!
Super Nutritious, Super Delicious Recipes

If you are reading this book, hopefully you have already had the chance to read *Intermittent Blasting - The Simple Truth Behind Consistently Losing Weight and Keeping It Off...For Good!* and learned the scientific principles of how and why our bodies use superfoods combined with intermittent fasting to lose weight, cleanse, and rejuvenate. This is a powerful combination and one that I feel will bring about a true revolution in our understanding of weight loss and overall health. We will touch on some of those concepts again here, but if you haven't read *Intermittent Blasting*, I encourage you to seek out a copy and introduce yourself to the concept of Intermittent Blasting and experience for yourself what it can do to create a healthier, more vibrant you.

The two most common questions I hear when speaking about Intermittent Blasting are: "What do I consume during an Intermittent Blast?" and "How do I transition back to normal eating after doing an Intermittent Blast?" These are both very important to consider when Intermittent Blasting, so I decided to devote an entire book to the subject. This book features:

- 50 smoothie recipes, some to be used during your Intermittent Blast and some to be used transitioning off your Intermittent Blast.
- 50 extremely nutrient-dense, easily digestible juice recipes that will Blast your body with focused nutrition during your Intermittent Blast.
- Nutrient-dense soup recipes to be enjoyed during and transitioning off your Intermittent Blast.

- Other recipes that are great for transitioning back to your normal diet. These are healthy snacks and meals that put you on a fast-track for health.
- Because quality nutrition is so important to your body every day, I included a brief discussion on the importance of Superfoods and what each one will do to help you maintain healthy weight and live a healthy life.
- Finally, this book would not be complete without a brief discussion on living a healthy life, cooking and shopping tips, and the importance of organic natural ingredients.

Chapter 2: Smoothies and Juicing

Intermittent Blasting Smoothies

Smoothies are a great addition to anyone's daily regimen. Smoothies are quick and simple to make, very convenient for those with a busy schedule, and there's no easier way to increase your daily servings of fruits and vegetables. Smoothies can be made ahead of time (the night before for example) and carried in a small cooler and can be consumed at your desk or even on the road.

The smoothie recipes included in chapter three are ideal to consume during an Intermittent Blast. Later in the book we will discuss other, more dense smoothies that you can try while transitioning to your normal diet (or anytime!). However, the ones in Chapter Three are ideal for consuming during your Intermittent Blast.

The key to making the healthiest, most delicious smoothies is to start with fresh, locally grown, organic produce. Most fruits and vegetables can be blended into a smoothie with the peel or rind on except citrus fruits such as oranges and grapefruit. There are obvious exceptions like bananas, pineapple and avocado. Pineapple can be juiced with the rind on but not blended into a smoothie and avocados must be peeled and seeded. Be creative and add any vegetables you crave and enjoy. Try to include vegetables (especially green vegetables) in every serving. Greens are rich in chlorophyll and are very alkalizing. Experiment by adding large handfuls of romaine, spinach, kale, Swiss chard, collard greens, bok choy, and any other dark green vegetables you can find locally and fresh. Also be sure to include healthy fats from whole food sources such as avocado, coconut oil and coconut butter. And on non-Intermittent Blasting days you can also add healthy protein from organic, free range eggs, high quality protein powders, and healthy fats from seeds and nuts.

Intermittent Blasting Recipes

Smoothies are actually very easy to make nowadays. If you don't want to go to the trouble of keeping fresh fruit and vegetables and cutting them up, you can buy frozen smoothie mixtures already pre-packaged. They even have large packages which contain individual bags of fruit for single serving smoothies. Once you have the fruits and vegetables you want to use all you need is a blender and your choice of liquid. You can make them ahead of time and store them in the refrigerator.

Juicing

Fresh cold-pressed juice is a great choice for your Intermittent Blast and can be taken alone or combined with whole food nutritional supplementation. Drinking just one fresh-pressed juice daily is a great way of Blasting your body with a wide variety of vitamins, minerals, and phytonutrients that can help you lose unwanted pounds and protect you against premature aging and disease. The challenge for most people is the time it takes to juice the produce and the expense of these nutritious beverages.

Let's address the issue of expense first. Ounce for ounce, we are talking about some of the very best nutrition on the planet. The fiber is pretty much all that is discarded in the process of juicing, so you are consuming highly concentrated gourmet liquid nutrition in a very easily digestible form. One 16-ounce glass of juice requires up to six pounds of fruits and vegetables, so it doesn't come cheap. But you have to consider the amount of nutrition rather than the sheer volume of food and you must keep in mind that investing in your health is one of the very best financial investments you will ever make. It is far cheaper to juice for a lifetime than to suffer a heart attack or be dependent on medication for a chronic condition that is totally avoidable.

Purchasing Fresh Cold-Pressed Juice

If it is impossible for you to make fresh juice yourself, or you would rather not inconvenience yourself, you do have additional options. Fortunately, there has been a recent surge in companies providing fresh, organic, cold-pressed juices. Movements such as ours are creating a demand for this kind of product. It's just a matter of logistics. If you live in a major metropolitan area, you will have no trouble finding a local company happy to supply you with fresh, organic cold-pressed beverages. However, if you live outside the larger cities, finding a local company providing this service may prove to be more difficult and you might have to consider purchasing from a vendor online. To locate companies providing these beverages you can simply conduct an Internet search using your local zip code along with "organic cold press juice". Just make sure their ingredients are fresh and organic and without preservatives. Juices made in this manner have a very short shelf life, so if a juice company promises you long storage times, look elsewhere.

How to Juice

Juicing does take a considerable amount of time, but it's well worth it. To make your own cold-pressed or slow-pressed juice, you will need a juicer or a combination of two separate machines. The type of juicer you will want to purchase is either a "cold press" or "slow press" juicer. These juice extraction methods are far superior to the more common centrifugal style juicer. Cold press or slow press methods allows for a much higher integrity of nutrients as no heat is used in the process. Almost all of the pulp is pressed out, which means less oxygen, which in turn gives a better-tasting, more nutritionally dense juice. Compared to the centrifugal juicing process, these juices are much higher in nutrition. In fact, it is estimated that cold-pressed juice contains three to five times more vitamins and minerals than fresh juice from a centrifugal juicer.

Intermittent Blasting Recipes

The gold standard of cold press juicers is the Norwalk and comes with a price tag of $2,500.00. A more economical way to produce fresh cold-pressed juice is to purchase a grinder (juicer with a grinding blade) and a juice press. The grinder will cost around $300.00-$500.00 and the press (Samson Welles Juice Press) is an additional $400.00. A simpler option is to purchase a slow juicer (which is known to produce similar quality juice as cold press juicers) and there are many options available on the market. Some do a better job of juicing harder produce, such as beets and carrots, while others do a better job with leafy greens, so there really is no single "best juicer". All things considered, I recommend the Hurom Slow Juicer or the Omega Vert, which are identical units. These juicers are practical, very efficient and can be purchased for around $300.00.

Great Juice Ingredients

The key to making the healthiest, most delicious juice is to start with fresh, locally grown, organic produce. If you have to choose between local and organic with the organic produce being shipped from a great distance, go with the fresher local produce. If you are unable to use organic vegetables and fruit, juicing is still well worthwhile, but be sure to wash the produce thoroughly.

Juicing Tips

Most fruits and vegetables can be juiced with the peel or rind on, except citrus fruits such as oranges and grapefruit. Lemons and limes are the exception and can be juiced with the rind on. For flavor you can add lemon, lime and/or ginger to most any juice. Be creative and add any vegetables you crave and enjoy.

It's always best to drink the juice immediately upon juicing as the nutrients begin to degrade with each passing minute. If necessary, you can store your freshly juiced beverages in the refrigerator for several days (the length of time will depend on the ingredients). If you decide to make enough juice for three or four days you can store your beverages in an airtight glass container in the refrigerator or you can even freeze your juice in the freezer. This is not ideal, but this juice is still much higher in nutrition than buying a common processed juice from the grocery.

Fresh-pressed juice is extremely rich in nutrition, but there is one thing you must always keep in mind. You want to consider the amount of sugar you are consuming when you drink juice as you want to avoid spiking your blood sugar level. The best way to achieve this is by using a higher ratio of vegetables (especially green vegetables) to fruits because fruit can be high in sugar. Greens are lower in carbohydrates and will not spike your blood sugar and insulin level, as sweeter fruits and vegetables can. Experiment by using large handfuls of romaine, spinach, kale, Swiss chard, collard greens, bok choy, and any other dark green vegetable you can find locally and fresh. You can also dilute the sugar content by adding water, or you can add healthy fats that slow digestion, like avocado, raw coconut or coconut oil, or soaked seeds such as chia or flax. Adding some fat from these healthy sources will also help to sustain and satiate you during your Intermittent Blast. When most people begin to consume juice, they prefer the sweeter juices because that's what they are used to consuming. As you get used to the healthier taste of vegetables, this will change and you will actually prefer beverages that are lower in sugar.

Benefits of Commonly Used Fruits and Vegetables in Smoothies and Juice

All fruits and vegetables provide a variety of health benefits, from building muscle and bones to cleansing the body of toxins. Below is a list of some of the many benefits of the most common fruits and vegetables used in juicing.

Apples

Apples are known to cleanse the gallbladder and liver. They are high in malic acid, which is said to play an important role in creating adenosine triphosphate (ATP). ATP is the body's primary source of energy at the cellular level. Apples also contain the potent detoxifying enzyme bromelain, which has cleansing, anti-inflammatory properties and cleanses the blood.

Beets

Beets are a wonderful tonic for the liver. Beets work as a cleanser for the bloodstream and are supportive of the heart and circulatory system in the body. Beets contain high amounts of boron, which is vital to the production of human sex hormones. Beets are full of potassium, magnesium, phosphorus, iron, vitamins A, B, & C, beta-carotene, beta-cyanine, and folic acid. Beets contain betaine, which is used in certain treatments of depression and also contains tryptophan, which relaxes the mind and creates a sense of well-being, similar to chocolate. Beets also contain folic acid which is necessary for the production of new cells. Beets contain the betalains betanin and vulgaxanthin. Both provide anti-inflammatory, antioxidant, and detoxification support.

Carrots

Carrots are packed with vitamins, minerals, and biotin, as well as powerful antioxidants, and also possess antimicrobial, antiviral, and anti-inflammatory properties, and aid blood circulation. Carrots are rich in vitamin A, which protects us from sun damage. Carrots have strong cleansing properties that are effective in detoxifying the liver, and very effective for treating acne that is caused by toxins in the blood. The vitamin A and other nutrients contained in carrots nourish the skin and prevent dry skin and other skin blemishes. Carrots are a great source of beta-carotene, which serves as an antioxidant that helps the body to fight against free radicals, is good for the eyes and also necessary for a shiny, well-moisturized hair and scalp. Beta-carotene also helps slow down the aging of cells and various negative effects associated with aging. Carrots are also high in potassium, an essential electrolyte necessary for cell function.

Celery

Truly a superfood, the simple celery plant provides an amazing number of important nutrients assisting many functions in the body. Celery is very alkalizing, highly nutritious, and is one of the most hydrating foods on the planet. The polyacetylene in celery is a powerful anti-inflammatory and the potassium and sodium in celery juice are powerful body-fluid regulators that stimulate urine production to help rid the body of excess fluid. Celery contains important concentrations of plant hormones and very special essential oils that give celery its characteristic smell. These oils help to regulate the nervous system and have a calming effect on the nervous system, making it beneficial for insomniacs. Its high magnesium levels help people to relax into a soothing and restful sleep. Celery juice is an amazing eliminator of toxins from the body, which aids in the breaking down and elimination of urinary and gallstones.

Cucumber

Cucumber is super-hydrating and charged with active enzymes, B vitamins, antioxidants, and electrolytes. Cucumbers are full of beautifying silica, as well as caffeic acid, which has anti-inflammatory properties. Cucumbers are extremely hydrating and are beneficial for the skin. Cucumbers have most of the vitamins the body needs in a single day. Due to its low calorie and high water content, the cucumber is an ideal food for people who are looking for weight loss. The high structured water content in cucumbers is very effective in ridding the body of toxins from the digestive system and is very alkalizing.

Lemons

Lemons are rich in the free-radical-fighting antioxidant vitamin C, and in flavonoids, which help to neutralize free radicals linked to aging and most diseases. Lemons improve blood flow and reduce inflammation. Though acidic to the taste, lemons are very alkalizing in the body. Lemons are a good source of electrolytes, such as potassium, calcium, and magnesium. Your liver loves lemons. Lemon is cleansing to the liver, causing toxins to be dumped by stimulating its natural enzymes, which helps keep skin even-toned and wrinkle-free. Lemons are a dissolvent of uric acid and other poisons, liquefy bile, and help dissolve gallstones, calcium deposits, and kidney stones. Lemons increase peristalsis, helping to eliminate waste. Lemons have powerful antibacterial properties; experiments have found the juice of lemons destroys the bacteria of malaria, cholera, diphtheria, typhoid, and other deadly diseases.

Kale

One of the healthiest vegetables on the planet, kale is in the brassica family which includes cruciferous vegetables such as cabbage, collards, broccoli, and brussels sprouts. Kale is a nutritional powerhouse packed with calcium, vitamin B6, magnesium, vitamin A, vitamin C, and vitamin K. It is also a good source of the minerals copper, potassium, iron, manganese, and phosphorus. Kale is rich in eye-health-promoting lutein and zeaxanthin. Per calorie, kale has more calcium than milk, which helps keep bones strong. Kale has more iron than beef, making it a great food for vegans and vegetarians. The vitamin A in kale is great for vision, skin, and nails. Kale is high in antioxidants such as carotenoids and flavonoids, is anti-inflammatory and extremely alkalizing. Amazingly, kale also has a healthy balance of omega-3 and omega-6 fatty acids.

Parsley

Parsley is much more than a decorative item placed on your plate to be discarded. Parsley is super-rich in antioxidants including luteolin, a flavonoid that eradicates free radicals in the body that cause oxidative stress in cells. Luteolin also promotes carbohydrate metabolism and is anti-inflammatory. Parsley is especially high in two powerful antioxidants, vitamins C and A, which serve to strengthen the body's immune system. Vitamin C is necessary for collagen production, the main structural protein found in connective tissue. This essential nutrient will not only accelerate the body's ability to repair wounds, but also maintain healthy bones and teeth. Vitamin A fortifies the entry points into the human body, such as mucus membranes, the lining of the eyes, and the respiratory, urinary and intestinal tracts. Furthermore, white blood cells rely on vitamin A to fight infection in the body. Parsley is also a great source of vitamin B12, vitamin K, beta carotene, folic acid and iron. Parsley (and greens in general) is a power-plant of chlorophyll, which is antibacterial and extremely alkalizing. Chlorophyll found in parsley is a good cure for bad breath. It also helps flush out excess fluid from the body, which supports kidney function.

Spinach

Spinach is an excellent source of vitamin K, vitamin A, magnesium, folate, manganese, iron, calcium, vitamin C, vitamin B2, potassium, vitamin B6, and a host of trace minerals. It's a very good source of protein, phosphorus, vitamin E, zinc, beta-carotene, and copper. And, it's a good source of selenium, niacin, and omega-3 fatty acids. The high amount of vitamin A in spinach promotes healthy skin by allowing for proper moisture retention in the epidermis, thus fighting psoriasis, keratinization, acne, and even wrinkles. Vitamin K in spinach promotes the synthesis of osteocalcin, the protein that is essential for maintaining the strength and density of our bones. It also contributes greatly to a healthy nervous system and brain function by providing an essential part of the synthesis of sphingolipids, the crucial fat that makes up the myelin sheath around our nerves. Spinach is loaded with flavonoids which act as antioxidants, protecting the body from free radicals. DNA damage and mutations in colon cells may be prevented by the folate that's present in spinach. In comparison to red meat, spinach provides a lot fewer calories, and is an excellent source of iron. Because iron is a component of hemoglobin, which carries oxygen to all body cells, it's needed for energy. Spinach is also anti-Inflammatory and very alkalizing.

As you can see, common everyday foods such as apples, beets, carrots, celery, cucumber, lemons, kale, parsley and spinach have tremendous powers for health and healing because they are packed with the nutrition we so desperately need. One of the best ways to get this nutrition in very concentrated form is by juicing. And one of the great things about juicing is that if you don't like something such as beets or kale for example, you can use juices such as apple, pineapple, lemon and ginger to offset the undesired taste and receive the benefits of the nutrition in a delicious beverage that you enjoy.

Chapter 3: Intermittent Blasting Recipes

Smoothies

Simple Smoothie

This is a smoothie I have been making for years. I vary it slightly depending on what's in season and I always use fresh, local, organic produce when possible.

- 1 cup blueberries
- 1/2 cup mango
- 1/2 avocado
- 1 small or 1/2 large apple
- 1 handful spinach
- Just enough water to mix

Additions for variety: Add peaches, strawberries or pineapple. For veggies, add raw or steamed carrots, cauliflower or a handful of greens of your choice. For protein, add raw, organic egg (from a trusted source) or protein from brown rice, hemp, pea or pumpkin seed. For fat/fiber, add soaked flax seeds or coconut butter. Substitute carrot juice or coconut water for water. **Add protein, seeds and nuts on non-Intermittent Blasting days only.**

Lemon Green

- 1 small apple
- 1/2 avocado
- 1 cucumber
- 2 cups spinach
- 2 large collard greens leaves
- 2 leaves black kale
- Juice of 3 lemons
- 1 1/2 cups water

Intermittent Blasting Recipes

Fruit and Salad Smoothie With Mint

- 1/2 cup water
- 1 apple cut into pieces
- 1 cup white grapes
- 1/3 cucumber, skinned and cut into pieces
- 2 lettuce leaves
- 1/2 stalk celery, cut into pieces
- 1 tablespoon fresh mint leaves
- 1/2 avocado

Strawberry Watermelon Smoothie

- 3 cups fresh watermelon cut into cubes
- 1 1/2 cups fresh strawberries
- A few fresh mint leaves to taste

Cut the watermelon into cubes and put in freezer for 2 hours or so as to be slightly frozen but not completely frozen. De-stem the strawberries. After washing the strawberries and mint leaves, blend all ingredients in blender until smooth. Add just enough water to blend.

Metal Detox

- 1/4 cup cilantro
- 1/4 cup parsley
- 1/4 cup dandelion greens
- 1/4 teaspoon pure organic chlorella powder
- 1/4 avocado
- 12 ounces filtered water

Fresh Almond Milk with Veggies and Berries

- 1/2 cup blueberries
- 1/2 cup blackberries
- 1/2 cup raspberries
- 1/2 cup strawberries
- 2 cups spinach

- 2 cups water
- 1/2 cup almonds

Put water and almonds (almonds can be soaked in water overnight if desired) into blender. Blend until you have almond milk (1-2 minutes). Add other ingredients and blend until smooth.

Green Tea Blast!

- 4 cups white grapes (frozen)
- 2 cups baby spinach (tightly packed)
- 1 and 1/2 cups brewed green tea
- 1/2 avocado
- Stevia or raw honey to taste

Brew green tea. Allow to cool. Blend ingredients until smooth.

Blueberry Piña Colada Blast

- 1/2 cup coconut milk
- 1/2 cup coconut water
- 1/4 small to medium pineapple or 3/4 cup frozen pineapple
- 1/2 cup blueberries
- 1/4 avocado
- 1 tablespoon shredded coconut

After removing the rind from the pineapple, cut into chunks. Remove peel and seed of avocado. Blend all ingredients with just enough water until smooth.

Raw Anti-Inflammatory Recovery Drink

- 6 cups red grapes
- 1 large carrot, not peeled
- 1 stalk celery
- 1" slice pineapple
- Just enough water to blend

Intermittent Blasting Recipes

Strawberry-Mango

- 8 ounces frozen strawberries
- 1/2 cup mango juice or sliced mango
- 1/4 avocado
- 1 tablespoon raw honey
- Just enough water to blend

Cherry Pomegranate

- 1/4 cup frozen sweet cherries
- 1/4 cup pomegranate-cherry juice
- 1/4 cup crushed pineapple in juice, drained, or fresh cut pineapple
- 1/4 banana, peeled and diced
- 1/4 avocado

Quick and Easy Smoothies (4 Ingredients or Less)

Delicious Kale Mango

- 3/4 cup mango
- 2 cups kale
- 1/2 avocado
- 1 1/2 cups coconut water

Mango Apple Blast

- 3/4 cup mango
- 3/4 cup apple
- 1/2 avocado
- 1 1/2 cups water

Mango Coconut Blast

- 3/4 cup mango
- 3/4 cup apple
- 2 tablespoons coconut oil
- 1 1/2 cups water

Intermittent Blasting Recipes

Training Smoothie

- 2 cups water
- 2 mangos, peeled
- 2 handfuls parsley
- Raw honey to taste

Electrolyte Grape-Ginger Lemonade

- 6 cups red grapes
- 1/4 lemon with peel
- 1 small slice ginger
- Just enough water to blend

Pineapple Blast

- 2 cups chopped pineapple (fresh or frozen)
- 1 cup pineapple juice, fresh-juiced if possible
- 1 1/2 cup coconut milk

After removing the rind from the pineapple, cut into chunks. Blend all ingredients until smooth.

Green Juices

These first juice recipes are green juices packed with vitamins, minerals (especially calcium), enzymes, chlorophyll, protein, electrolytes, and phytonutrients. Green juices in particular are amazing for energy, muscle recovery and detoxification and are extremely alkalizing.

If you are not accustomed to the taste of green juice you may prefer to increase the amounts of sweeter juices such as apple, pineapple, pear and mango. For a thicker, creamier beverage add 1/4 - 1/2 avocado (peeled and pitted) and/or 1 tablespoon coconut oil and blend in a blender.

Newbie Green

This is a delicious green drink designed for those who might not be ready for the really green goodness just yet.

- 4 medium apples
- 4 stalks celery
- 1 cucumber
- 1 very small piece of ginger root to taste (1/8 inch or so)
- 1/2 lemon
- 1 peeled orange
- 1 large handful spinach

Simple Green

- 2 apples: Granny Smith, Gala or Golden Delicious if possible
- 1 cucumber
- 1 bunch kale
- 4 stalks celery
- 1/2 lemon including skin

Greens with Carrot

- 4 carrots
- 1 cucumber
- 1-2 cups spinach
- 1 lemon
- 1/2 bunch dandelion greens
- 1 apple; Green, Gala or Pink Lady
- 1 pear

Green Lemonade

- 3 cups spinach
- 1 lemon
- 1 cucumber
- 1 pear
- 1 apple; Green, Gala or Pink Lady

Intermittent Blasting Recipes

Greens with Pea Sprouts

- 2 large cucumbers
- 4 celery stalks
- Large handful kale
- Large handful of sweet pea sprouts
- 1-2 broccoli stems
- 1 green apple
- 1/2 inch piece of ginger (add more if you want your juice to have a kick to it)

Optional additions or substitutions: Dandelion greens, romaine, parsley, spinach.

Green Detox

- 1/2 small head of dark green lettuces such as green leaf lettuces, romaine, endives
- Handful dandelion greens
- 3 leaves beet tops
- 6 leaves watercress
- 3 leaves red cabbage
- 1/4 green bell pepper
- Small handful of Swiss chard
- 1 green apple

Dr. Oz's Green Drink

This is a recipe Dr. Mehmet Oz is said to drink every morning.

- 2 medium apples
- 3 stalks celery
- 1 cucumber
- 12 grams ginger root (just a pinch)
- 1/2 lemon
- 1 medium lime
- 1 bunch parsley
- 2 cups spinach

Greens and Berries

- 4 leaves romaine lettuce
- 4 leaves kale
- 4 leaves endive
- 1 handful spinach
- 2 stalks celery
- 2 broccoli stems
- 1 cucumber
- 6 strawberries
- 2 basil leaves

Coconut Green

- 2 cups coconut water (fresh if possible)
- 1 bunch kale
- 1 handful spinach
- 5 stalks celery
- 1 medium apple of your choice
- 1/2 bunch parsley
- 1 small lemon

Greens With A Kick

- 2 cucumbers
- 1 bunch spinach
- 1/2 bunch kale
- 1 bunch cilantro
- 2 limes
- Jalapeño to taste

Veggies and Greens

- 4 medium carrots
- 3 stalks celery
- 1 medium to large cucumber
- 1/2 bunch kale
- 1/2 bunch cilantro

Intermittent Blasting Recipes

- 1/2 bunch parsley
- 1 handful spinach
- 1 small lemon

Greens with Ginger

- 2 green apples
- 2 pears
- 1/2 inch fresh ginger
- 1 lemon
- 2 stalks kale
- 1/2 bunch dandelion greens
- 1 handful spinach

Super Liver Support

- 8 large carrots
- 8 dandelion green leaves
- 2 medium beets
- 2 medium apples
- 1 small piece of ginger

Beets and Greens

- 2 medium beets
- 2 medium to large apples
- 5 radishes
- 3 stalks kale
- 1 handful spinach

Delicious Green Tea

- 2 medium apples
- 6 medium carrots
- 12 ounces green tea
- 1 and 1/2 teaspoon raw honey
- 1/4 lemon
- 1 small orange (peeled)

Intermittent Blasting Recipes

Brew 12 ounces of green tea, add honey to taste. While allowing tea to cool to room temperature, juice the other ingredients. Mix together and enjoy!

Quick and Easy Juices (4 Ingredients or Less)

These juices do not require a lot of time or ingredients to prepare, so they are perfect for an active, busy lifestyle. Many of these quick recipes pack as big a nutritional punch as the others and require half the time to prepare. These recipes can also be transformed into smoothies by simply using the whole fruit (peeled and pitied when appropriate) and adding liquid such as water or nut milk and blend in a blender.

Greens and Grapefruit

- 15 large kale leaves
- Handful dandelion greens
- 2 large pink grapefruits, peeled
- 8 leaves of mint

Fruit Peppermint

- 1/2 pineapple
- 1 medium apple
- 1 cup strawberries
- 15 leaves peppermint

Watermelon Cucumber with Mint

- 8 cups diced watermelon
- 1 large cucumber
- Handful (about 15 or so) mint leaves
- 1 lime

Apple Strawberry

- 3 large apples
- 5 cups strawberries

Intermittent Blasting Recipes

- 1 large carrot
- 1/2 lime

Orange Pineapple Blast

- 1 large or 2 small oranges
- 1/4 pineapple
- 3 medium carrots
- 1/4-1/2 small to medium lemon

Be sure to remove the rind from the orange.

Liver Cleanse

- 1 large or 2 small apples of your choice
- 1 large or 2 small beets
- 3 large or 4 medium carrots

This particular combination is terrific for cleansing the liver, lowers inflammation, aids blood circulation, and is packed with potassium, magnesium, phosphorus, iron, vitamins A, B & C, beta-carotene, beta-cyanine, folic acid, and biotin. This juice has antimicrobial, antiviral, anti-aging, anti-inflammatory powers and antioxidants that help the body fight free radicals.

LemonAid

- 8 apples
- 1/2 lemon

This LemonAid is simple, delicious and very nutritious. It is a great source of antioxidants, flavonoids, and electrolytes, is anti-inflammatory, antibacterial and cleanses the blood. This drink will help cleanse the liver and gallbladder, increase energy, and is alkalizing.

Pineapple Mango

- 1 large pineapple
- 1 large mango

Intermittent Blasting Recipes

Quick Apple Strawberry

- 2 medium apples
- 12 medium carrots
- 1.5 cups strawberries

Quick Carrot Apple

- 10 medium carrots
- 3 medium apples

Beet Apple Blast!

- 2 beets
- 2 medium apples
- 1/2 inch slice ginger

Quick Apple Pear

- 5 medium apples
- 2 pears

Apple Carrot with Ginger

- 2 green apples
- 10 medium carrots
- 1 handful spinach
- 1/2 inch slice ginger

Carrot Spinach with Kale

- 10 carrots
- 2 handfuls spinach
- 2 leaves kale

Strawberry Watermelon Blast

- 1/4 medium to large watermelon
- 15 medium strawberries
- 1 large apple

Carrots with Greens

- 6 medium to large carrots

Intermittent Blasting Recipes

- 1 handful spinach
- 4 sprigs parsley
- 5 kale leaves

Cabbage, Celery, Lime

- 1 head red or green cabbage
- 7 medium stalks celery
- 2 limes

Apple, Celery, Cucumber

- 4 medium apples
- 2 celery stalks
- 1 small cucumber

Romaine, Celery, Apple

- 12 leaves romaine lettuce
- 4 stalks celery
- 2 apples of your choice

Celery, Carrot, Apple

- 8 medium stalks celery
- 5 large carrots
- 2 apples of your choice

Pineapple Strawberry

- 1/2 pineapple
- 12-15 strawberries

Carrot Cucumber Beet

- 8 carrots
- 1 medium cucumber
- 1 small to medium beet

Carrot Beet Parsley

- 10 medium carrots
- 1 small beet

Intermittent Blasting Recipes

- 5 sprigs parsley

Romaine, Cabbage, Carrot
- 10 leaves romaine lettuce
- 4 cups green cabbage
- 5 medium carrots

Carrot, Apple, Potato (yes, potato)
- 2 carrots
- 2 apples
- 2 potatoes (with peel)
- Add lemon, lime or ginger to taste, if desired.

Dinner Juices

These juices can be consumed anytime, but some people enjoy these more savory beverages later in the day. They do pack a huge amount of nutrition, so I encourage you to try at least one or two during your Intermittent Blast.

Healthy Veggie (V-8)
- 2 large carrots
- 3 stalks celery
- 1 medium beet
- 1/2 cucumber
- 1 handful parsley
- 1/2 medium green pepper
- 1 cup spinach
- 3 medium tomatoes

V3 with Lemon
- 2 tomatoes
- 3 stalks celery
- 1 carrot
- Sliver of lemon

Intermittent Blasting Recipes

V4

- 10 leaves romaine lettuce
- 2 medium tomatoes
- 2 stalks celery
- 4 medium carrots

Kale, Carrots, Celery

- 1 bunch kale
- 4 carrots
- 4 stalks celery

Asparagus Juice

- 6 spears asparagus
- 4 large carrots
- 3 stalks celery

It's not as bad as it sounds. And it's very healthy!

Carrot, Celery, Romaine

- 2 medium carrots
- 2 stalks celery
- 6 leaves romaine lettuce

Carrot, Parsley, Romaine, Lemon

- 2 medium carrots
- Handful parsley
- 6 leaves romaine lettuce
- 1 sliver lemon

Swiss Chard, Carrot, Celery

- Large bunch Swiss chard
- 2 medium carrots
- 2 stalks celery

Salsa Fresh

- 2 stalks celery

Intermittent Blasting Recipes

- 2 handfuls cilantro
- 1 medium spring onion
- 2 cloves garlic
- 2 small green peppers
- Cayenne pepper to taste (a dash or two)
- 2 medium tomatoes

Salt to taste (Celtic Sea Salt, Himalayan, Real Salt or Aztec sea salt).

Blast O' Veggies

- 4 tomatoes
- 2 green onions
- 1/2 green pepper
- 2 stalks celery
- 2 medium carrots
- Handful cilantro
- Handful parsley
- Handful spinach
- 1/2 lemon

Salt to taste (Celtic Sea Salt, Himalayan, Real Salt or Aztec sea salt).

Soups

These simple and nutritious soups are great for adding variety to your Intermittent Blast and are helpful for those who miss the sensation of "eating". Each recipe makes about 2 servings.

Creamy Broccoli

- 2 cups vegetable stock (Imagine or Pacific for example)
- 4 cups broccoli, chopped
- 2 yellow onions, chopped

Intermittent Blasting Recipes

- 1 red bell pepper, chopped
- 2 stalks celery, chopped
- 1 avocado
- Salt, pepper, soy sauce or Bragg's Liquid Aminos to taste

Put all ingredients except the avocado in blender and blend until smooth. Add the avocado and blend on low speed until smooth. Add more or less stock or water to create the desired consistency. Transfer to pot, warm and serve.

Tomato Basil

- 3 medium tomatoes, diced
- 4 slices sun-dried tomato
- 2 medium stalks celery, diced
- 1 pinch onion powder
- 1 pinch garlic powder
- 1 pinch dried basil or 2 sprigs of fresh basil
- 1/2 avocado
- Salt and pepper to taste

Put the tomatoes and sun-dried tomatoes into the blender and blend until smooth. Add the rest of the ingredients except the avocado and blend for 1 minute or until smooth. Add water if needed. Add the avocado and lightly blend on low until smooth.

Raw Creamy Cucumber Avocado

- 2 medium cucumbers
- 2 avocados
- 1/2 cup fresh lemon juice
- 3 cloves garlic, peeled and minced
- 1 cup cilantro, finely chopped
- 1 cup of water
- 2 teaspoons salt

Put all ingredients except the avocado in blender and blend until smooth. Add the avocado and blend on low speed until smooth. Add more or less stock or water to create the desired consistency. Serve chilled.

Super Green

- 1 cup vegetable stock (Imagine or Pacific for example)
- 2 medium cucumbers
- 1 cup spinach
- 1 medium onion
- 1 clove garlic, peeled and minced
- 1/2 red bell pepper
- 1 avocado
- 1/2 teaspoon curry powder
- Lime juice to taste
- Salt, pepper, soy sauce or Bragg's Liquid Aminos to taste

Put all ingredients except the avocado in blender and blend until smooth. Add the avocado and blend on low speed until smooth. Add more or less stock or water to create the desired consistency. Transfer to pot and warm.

Raw Almond Pea Soup

- 2 cups green peas
- 1 avocado
- 1 1/2 cups almond milk (freshly made if possible)
- 1/2 medium onion
- 1 teaspoon salt to taste
- 1/2 teaspoon pepper to taste

Put all ingredients except the avocado in blender and blend until blended well. Add the avocado and blend on low speed until smooth.

Creamed Spinach Soup

- 2 cups baby spinach leaves, washed thoroughly
- 1/2 cucumber, peeled
- 1 medium tomato, diced

Intermittent Blasting Recipes

- 1 avocado
- 1/4 cup water
- 1 clove garlic, peeled and minced
- 2 tablespoon soy sauce or Bragg's Aminos
- 1 tablespoon olive oil
- 1 tablespoon lemon juice
- 1 pinch cayenne pepper
- 1/2 teaspoon salt or to taste
- Black pepper to taste

Put all ingredients except the avocado in blender and blend until blended well. Add the avocado and blend on low speed until smooth.

Watermelon Mango Soup

- 5 cups diced watermelon
- 2 cups mango, peeled and diced (fresh or frozen)
- 1/4 cup lime juice (fresh if possible)
- Handful fresh mint, finely chopped
- 1/4 avocado
- 2 teaspoons fresh ginger, minced
- 1 tablespoon raw honey
- Two pinches freshly ground cardamom

Put all ingredients except the avocado in blender and blend until blended well. Add the avocado and blend on low speed until smooth. Chill in refrigerator for two hours.

Optional. You can hold out about 1/4 to 1/3 of the watermelon and mango and add after blending for a chunkier feel.

Avocado Mint

- 2 1/2 cups water
- 1 avocado
- 1 small cucumber, peeled and diced
- 1 handful mint leaves

Intermittent Blasting Recipes

- 1 handful spinach
- 1 small clove garlic, peeled and minced
- 2 tablespoons fresh lime juice
- 1 tablespoon salt to taste
- Black pepper to taste

Put all ingredients except the avocado in blender and blend until blended well. Add the avocado and blend on low speed until smooth. Add water if needed to blend.

Raw Sweet Potato Soup

- 1 medium sweet potato, peeled and diced
- 1 pear
- 1/2 medium banana
- 1/4 teaspoon cinnamon
- 1/2 avocado
- 1 cup almond milk, fresh if possible
- 1/4 teaspoon pumpkin spice
- 3 dates, pitted
- 1 cup hot water

Put all ingredients except the avocado in blender and blend until blended well. Add the avocado and blend on low speed until smooth. Add water if needed to blend.

Raw Green Veggie Soup

- 5 handfuls spinach
- 1 handful fresh cilantro
- 2-3 sprigs of fresh parsley
- 3 slices green pepper
- 1 tablespoon raw onion, finely diced
- 1 small clove garlic, peeled and minced
- 1 small zucchini, diced
- 2 stalks celery, diced
- 1 avocado

Intermittent Blasting Recipes

- 1/4 cup almonds, soaked overnight and rinsed
- 1 1/2 cups water
- 1/2 lemon juiced
- Salt to taste

Put ingredients except the avocado in blender and blend until blended well. Add the avocado and blend on low speed until smooth. Add water if needed to blend. Warm on low heat or until just warm and serve.

Chapter 4: After The Intermittent Blast

People often ask how to best transition to their normal diet following their Intermittent Blast. When you put your body into a mode of cleansing for a 2-day stretch or longer, it's best not to immediately dive into a steak dinner with all the fixings. Those who make that mistake are not likely to repeat it again as the effect it has on the body can be quite dramatic. If you were not aware of this, then please understand that after a period of resting the digestive tract (Intermittent Blast), you need to take a bit more care with what you eat so your body can adjust back into a digesting mode easily and comfortably. This should only take 12 - 24 hours. Here are some ideal recipes to consider when transitioning between Intermittent Blasting and eating normally.

Transitional Smoothies

These smoothies can be enjoyed every day or as a quick and delicious way to transition back to your normal diet following an Intermittent Blast. They require a little more energy from the digestive tract, so they are not ideal to be used while Blasting.

Fruit Smoothie 101

- 1 cup fresh or frozen berries and any other fresh fruit of your choice
- 1/2 apple
- 1 tablespoon soaked or powdered flax seeds
- 1/2 avocado
- Enough filtered water to blend

Banana Berry

- 1 medium banana
- 6 strawberries
- Handful spinach
- 1 tablespoon cinnamon

Intermittent Blasting Recipes

- Flax seed milk or almond milk (just enough to blend)

Coconut Milk Pina Colada

- 1 cup chopped pineapple (fresh or frozen)
- 1 cup coconut milk
- 1/2 cup pineapple juice
- 1/4 avocado
- 1 large banana
- 1 cup spinach (raw or steamed)
- 2 tablespoons dried coconut
- 1 teaspoon vanilla extract or vanilla bean, to taste

Strawberry Coconut

- 1 cup coconut milk
- 1 medium banana
- 2 cups strawberries (fresh or frozen)
- 1 teaspoon vanilla extract or vanilla bean, to taste

Blueberry Coconut Smoothie

- 1/2 cup coconut milk
- 1/2 cup coconut water or water
- 1 large banana
- 1 cup blueberries (fresh or frozen)
- 2 tablespoon dried coconut (optional)
- 1 tablespoon raw almonds
- 1/4 avocado

Fruit Salad with Mint

- 1 apple cut in pieces
- 1 cup white grapes
- 1/3 cucumber, peeled and cut in large pieces
- 2 lettuce leaves
- 1/2 stick celery, cut into pieces
- 1 tablespoon fresh mint leaves
- 1/2 cup water

Intermittent Blasting Recipes

Banana Lime Cinnamon

- 1 medium banana
- Juice of 1/2 lime
- 1/2 cup fresh or frozen raspberries
- 1 teaspoon maca powder
- 1 pinch cinnamon
- 1 cup filtered water

Coconut Kale Blast!

- 1/2 cup coconut water
- 1/4 cup coconut milk
- 1 cup kale (chopped)
- 1 medium banana
- 1/2 cup mango (fresh or frozen)
- 1/2 avocado
- Stevia or raw honey, to taste (optional)

Delicious Chocolate Blast!

- 1 medium frozen banana cut into slices
- 1/2 avocado
- 2 tablespoons raw cacao powder
- 1 tablespoon raw honey
- 1 cup coconut or almond milk

Healthy Chocolate Banana Blast!

- 1 small banana
- 1 tablespoon raw cacao powder
- 1 teaspoon maca powder
- 1 cup almond milk
- 1/4 cup coconut milk
- Salt and cinnamon to taste

Peel banana and blend all ingredients until smooth.

Intermittent Blasting Recipes

Creamy Coconut Strawberry Blast!

- 1 cup strawberries
- 1 cup coconut milk
- 1 cup coconut water from a young coconut
- 1 cup coconut meat from a young coconut
- 1 tablespoon coconut oil
- 1/2 small avocado
- Stevia or raw honey to taste

Banana Berry Fruit Smoothie

- 1 medium banana
- 6 strawberries
- Flax seed milk or almond milk
- Handful spinach
- 1 tablespoon cinnamon

Chocolate Almond Banana Blast

- 1 cup chocolate almond milk
- 1 medium banana
- 2 tablespoons organic natural almond butter (or other nut butter)
- 1 tablespoon ground flaxseed
- 1 tablespoon coconut oil
- Piña Colada
- 1/2 cup coconut milk
- 1/2 cup pineapple-coconut juice
- 1/2 small banana
- 1/2 apple
- 1 teaspoon raw coconut or unsweetened dry coconut
- 1/3 cup fresh or frozen pineapple

The Banana Berry

- 1 banana
- 6 strawberries
- Almond or Flaxseed milk

Intermittent Blasting Recipes

- Handful spinach leaves
- 1 tablespoon cinnamon

Cranberry-Green Tea

- 1/2 cup frozen cranberries
- 1/4 cup blueberries
- 1/2 cup blackberries
- 5 medium strawberries
- 1 medium banana, chopped into chunks
- 1/2 cup brewed green tea, cooled to room temperature
- 1/4 cup plain almond, hemp, or oat milk
- 2 tablespoons raw honey

For a more tropical smoothie, substitute coconut milk for the almond, hemp, or oat milk and add one cup frozen pineapple chunks and a tablespoon of fresh raw coconut instead of the blackberries and strawberries.

Banana Peach

- 1 medium banana
- 1/2 cup fresh (or frozen without sugar) peaches
- 1 cup almond, hemp, or oat milk

Strawberry Banana

- 2 cups strawberries (fresh or frozen)
- 2 medium bananas
- 4 tablespoon coconut milk
- 1 teaspoon lemon juice
- 1 1/2 cup coconut water or water

Coconut Banana

- 16 ounces coconut milk
- 2 medium bananas
- 1 tablespoon ground flaxseed, sunflower and pumpkin seed
- 1 mango, diced, or 1 cup frozen mango chunks

Intermittent Blasting Recipes

- 1/2 avocado

Blueberry Mango Blast

- 1 cup frozen blueberries
- 1 cup mango chunks
- 1/2 avocado
- 1/4 cup almond milk, or just enough to blend

Banana Cream Pie

- 1/2 cup sliced banana
- 1/4 cup almond milk
- 1/4 avocado
- 1 tablespoon whole wheat graham cracker crumbs
- 1/4 teaspoon natural vanilla extract

Freeze banana slices in a single layer on a baking sheet, and freeze until firm (about 1 hour). Place frozen banana and remaining ingredients in a blender and blend until smooth, adding more almond milk if needed. Sprinkle with additional graham cracker crumbs if desired.

Blackberry-Mango

- 3/8 cup fresh or frozen blackberries
- 1/4 cup chilled or frozen mango slices
- 1/4 avocado
- 1/4 cup orange juice
- 2 teaspoons raw honey

Optional: Blueberries can be substituted for blackberries.

Strawberry-Banana

- 1 1/2 cups fresh or frozen strawberries
- 1 banana, chopped in chunks
- 3/8 cup almond milk
- 1/2 avocado
- 1/8 cup raw honey

Vanilla Fruit

- 1/2 cup almond milk
- 1/8 cup pineapple-orange juice
- 1/2 cup fresh or frozen strawberries
- 1/2 banana, chopped into chunks

Substitute different fruits (such as cherries, blueberries, pineapple, etc.) if desired.

Jump-Start your Day!

- 1/2 cup orange juice
- 4 to 6 fresh or frozen strawberries
- 1/2 banana
- 1/4 avocado
- 1 tablespoon raw honey

Pineapple Kale

- 1/2 cup coconut milk
- 1 cup raw or lightly steamed kale or spinach
- 1 1/2 cups chopped pineapple (about 1/4 medium pineapple)
- 1 medium banana
- 1/2 cup water or just enough to make smooth

Hot-Spot Smoothie Recipes

Longevity Hot Spots are places throughout the world where people live longer and healthier lives. The following smoothie recipes are inspired by various Longevity Hot Spots and contain specific ingredients credited with aiding their incredible health in that particular area of the world.

The Okinawa Tropical

- 1 banana
- 1/2 papaya

- 1/2 fresh mango or 1/2 cup frozen mango chunks
- 1 cup almond milk
- 2 tablespoons dried organic coconut

The Symi Minty Green

- 1/2 cup water
- 1 apple, cut into pieces
- 1 cup white grapes
- 1/3 cucumber skinned and cut in large pieces
- 1/2 stalk celery, cut in pieces
- 1 tablespoon fresh mint leaves

The Campodimele Tomato and Herb

- 1 cup tomato juice
- 2 tablespoons fresh parsley
- 1 teaspoon dried mixed herbs (thyme, sage, basil, etc.)
- 1/2 cup fennel
- 1 stalk celery
- 1 shallot or half a small onion
- 1 small carrot
- 1/2 cup cucumber
- Juice of 1 lemon

The Sardinia Red Grape

- 1/2 cup red grape juice
- 1 cup seedless red grapes
- 1 cup raspberries
- 1 cup almond milk

The Nicoya Avocado

- 1 avocado
- A few slices Gala apple (optional)
- 1 cucumber
- 2 cups spinach
- 2 large leaves collard greens

- 2 leaves black kale
- juice of 3 lemons
- 1 1/2 cups water

The Loma Linda Nut and Cinnamon

- 1 cup almond milk
- 1/2 cup chopped dates
- 3 tablespoons ground almonds, hazelnuts, pecans, or macadamia nuts
- 1 banana
- 1 large pinch cinnamon
- 1 small pinch ground nutmeg

The Hunza Apricot

- 1 cup almond, hemp, or oat milk
- 1 cup chopped soft organic apricots (soften first by soaking in hot water, if necessary)
- 1 heaped tablespoon ground flax seeds
- 1 heaped tablespoon ground almonds or apricot kernels
- 1 banana

The Bama Exotic Fruit

- 1/2 cup almond, hemp, or oat milk
- 1 guava
- 1 pear
- 1 banana

Transitional Soups

Soups are an ideal way to ease back into your normal diet following an Intermittent Blast. They can pack a nutritious punch while easing your digestion processes back on. Try some of the following recipes and experiment with your favorite vegetables – chop them up with onion and garlic, sweat them in olive oil or coconut oil, add stock and simmer until the vegetables are soft. You can even blend them in the blender if you like.

Intermittent Blasting Recipes

Bone Broth / Bone Marrow Soup

Consuming bone broth is one of the best things you can do to improve and maintain great health. Bone broth has been used by physicians as far back as Hippocrates' day, is used today by holistic physicians, and is a staple throughout longevity societies. It is known to improve digestion and mental health, alleviate allergies, strengthen the immune system, and is a great remedy for the cold and flu. Rich in minerals, bone broth is also known to improve connective tissue and even re-mineralize teeth. Thanks to the gelatin in the broth, it's great for healthy hair and nail growth and can even eliminate cellulite. Bone broth probably gives the best bang for the buck when it comes to nutrition because it is very affordable to produce. You can take it alone by sipping throughout the day, or you can use it as a base for soup.

Bones: When it comes to bones, the rule of thumb is the larger the better, as the larger bones have more marrow than smaller bones. Ideally you can use large beef marrow and knuckle bones and short rib bones, but in a pinch a chicken carcass will do.

Ideal example:

- 6 pounds of bones (beef marrow, knuckle bones, short ribs). Always use bones from organically grown animals
- 1/2 cup raw apple cider vinegar
- 4 quarts filtered water

Place bones in large pot or crockpot and pour in water and vinegar and let sit for an hour or so. Add water if necessary to cover. Bring to boil and skim the foam from the top. Reduce heat, cover, and simmer for at least 24 hours and up to three days, adding water occasionally. Consider turning heat off overnight and heat back to a low simmer in the morning. Let sit and cool and then strain. The bones can be broken to insure the excretion of the marrow. Over the last hour or so you can add vegetables such as celery, carrots, onions and salt. Broth can be stored in the refrigerator for up to a week or in the freezer for up to six months.

Simple Veggie Soup

- 2 cloves garlic, peeled and minced
- 1 small onion, peeled and diced
- 1/4 green bell pepper, diced
- 1/4 red bell pepper, diced
- 3 medium carrots, diced
- 1/2 cup Brussels sprouts
- 4 medium potatoes, diced
- 1/4 cup green peas
- 1/4 cup black-eyed peas
- 1/4 cup kidney beans
- 1/4 cup lentils
- 2 cups tomato juice
- 32 ounces bone broth, or organic vegetable broth (Imagine or Pacific, for example)
- Salt, pepper and spices of choice, to taste

If you are using un-prepped (raw) beans, lentils, and peas, they should be soaked in water overnight.

Start by sweating the onion, garlic, and peppers in a heavy cast-iron skillet with coconut oil, olive oil, or red palm oil until soft. Transfer to a large pot filled with a couple of cups of tomato juice and 32 ounces of bone broth, or organic vegetable broth (Imagine, 365, or Pacific, for example). Cook on medium to high heat until the soup reaches a boil and lower heat to medium-low. After prepping the additional ingredients (washing all produce thoroughly, and dicing the potatoes and carrots), add everything to the pot except the potatoes. Cook on medium heat for thirty to forty minutes, then add the potatoes. Continue to cook an additional twenty minutes until potatoes are soft throughout. Take pot off heat and serve.

Intermittent Blasting Recipes

Ratatouille

- 1 medium/large sweet or yellow onion, peeled and diced
- 4 cloves garlic, minced
- 2 green or red bell peppers (or one of each), diced or sliced into 1/2" strips
- 4 large tomatoes, peeled and diced
- 2 medium zucchini, sliced in 1/2" pieces
- 3 small eggplants, cut in 1" pieces
- 2 teaspoons of dried thyme
- 1/8 cup finely chopped fresh basil
- 6 tablespoons olive oil
- 2 tablespoon chopped parsley
- 1/2 cup tomato juice
- 1/2 cup water
- 2 teaspoons salt
- Black pepper

Don't peel the vegetables other than the eggplant, garlic and onion. Cook onion in olive oil over medium/low heat until soft, 5-7 minutes. Add garlic and cook an additional minute or two. Add the water, tomato juice, and peppers and cook until peppers are soft, about 6-8 minutes. Add the rest of the ingredients and cook covered for about 45 minutes stirring occasionally. Increase or decrease the water and tomato juice depending on the desired consistency. Add salt and pepper to taste.

Leek, Potato, and Watercress

- 1 leek, chopped
- 1 potato, chopped
- 1 bunch watercress
- 1/2 tablespoon butter
- 2 tablespoons olive oil
- Chicken stock or vegetable stock
- Lemon juice

Intermittent Blasting Recipes

- Salt and freshly ground black pepper to taste

Heat the butter and olive oil on medium/low heat in a heavy-based pan. Add the potato and gently cook for 5-10 minutes. Add the leek, put a lid on the pan, and sweat the vegetables for an additional 5-10 minutes, stirring occasionally. Add enough stock to cover the vegetables – you can cover with water and add stock in cube form if you don't have real stock. Add more water or stock if you like your soup thinner. Simmer with a lid on until the vegetables are soft. Add the watercress, and simmer for 3 minutes. Serve or blend in blender if you like and serve. Squeeze in lemon juice and add salt and pepper to taste.

Zucchini Soup

- 3 zucchinis, cut into 1 inch pieces
- 2 tablespoons olive oil or coconut oil
- 1-2 garlic cloves, chopped small or minced
- Chicken stock or vegetable stock
- 4-5 basil leaves, torn into smaller pieces
- A small bunch flat-leaf parsley, chopped
- Salt and freshly ground black pepper, to taste

Heat the oil on medium-low heat in a heavy-based pan. Add the zucchinis and garlic and sweat or cook gently until the zucchinis are soft – this will take about 25 minutes. Add enough stock or water to cover the vegetables and simmer for a few minutes. Blend around three-quarters of the soup until pureed and return to the pan with the rest. Add salt and a grind or two of pepper, herbs. Stir and serve.

Tomato Soup

This delicious soup is full of lycopene and can be served either warm or chilled.

- 1 pound ripe tomatoes, quartered
- 1 small onion, diced
- 1 carrot, diced

Intermittent Blasting Recipes

- 1 clove garlic, chopped finely or minced
- 1/4 teaspoon dried thyme
- 1/4 teaspoon dried marjoram
- 1 small bay leaf
- 1 tablespoon olive oil
- Salt and freshly-ground pepper to taste

Bring water to a boil in a saucepan, remove from the heat, and put the tomatoes in the water. Remove after 1 minute and peel off the skins. Heat the olive oil on low to medium heat in a heavy-based pan. Add the onion and carrot and cook for 3-4 minutes until slightly softened. Add the tomatoes, garlic, herbs, salt, and pepper. Simmer on medium-low heat with a lid on for 30 minutes. Remove and discard the bay leaf and blend the soup. Serve.

Quick Bean and Tomato Soup

This simple recipe makes a very sustaining soup and is perfect with a salad. If you are busy and don't want to spend time making lunch, you can make it in batches and freeze it, then heat it up when you are ready to eat it. If you want to eat it in the office or on the road and have no cooking facilities, it is worth investing in a food flask so you can heat it up in the morning and have it at lunch time.

- 1 can beans or 2-3 cups soaked and cooked beans (kidney beans, aduki beans, and black beans work well)
- 2 large peeled tomatoes or 1 can tomatoes
- 2 tablespoons olive oil
- 2 tablespoons butter (optional)
- 1 onion, diced
- 1-2 cloves garlic, minced
- 1 stalk celery, chopped
- 1 cube organic chicken or vegetable stock
- 1/2 cup water
- 1 teaspoon mixed herbs
- A wedge of lemon

Intermittent Blasting Recipes

- Salt and pepper, to taste

Heat the olive oil and butter on medium-low heat in a heavy-based pan. Add the onion, celery, and garlic and cook gently for about 5-10 minutes until soft. Add the canned tomatoes, stock cube, and water and simmer with the lid on for about 10 minutes, making sure to stir the stock cube in well. Add the beans, herbs, and seasoning, and more water if needed, and simmer with the lid on for another 5 minutes. Blend to the desired consistency and serve with the squeeze of lemon. Add salt and pepper, to taste.

Mung Bean Soup

Mung beans, a traditional food in China and in Okinawa, are a great source of protein, fiber, and folate. In China, they are used to treat food poisoning, mumps, and skin conditions; they are considered to have powerful detoxifying properties in Ayurvedic medicine.

- 3 cups mung beans, soaked overnight and cooked
- 2 tablespoons olive oil
- 1 onion, finely chopped
- 1 carrot, finely chopped
- 1 stalk celery, finely chopped
- 1 teaspoon fresh ginger ground, dried or minced
- 1/2 teaspoon ground coriander seeds
- 1/2 teaspoon ground cumin
- 1 teaspoon turmeric
- 1 lemon
- 1 tablespoon cilantro, finely chopped
- Salt and pepper

Heat the olive oil on medium-low heat in a heavy-based pan and add the onion. Stir for 2-3 minutes. Then add the carrot, celery, coriander seeds, ginger, and cumin. Stir for another 5 minutes. Then add water or stock to amply cover the vegetables (how much depends on how thin you like your soup) and simmer with a lid on for around

40 minutes, or until the carrots are soft. Add the mung beans and turmeric, heat through, and serve with a squeeze of lemon, and cilantro. Add salt and pepper, to taste.

Gazpacho

Make this soup when the vegetables are in season – try to get vine-ripened organic tomatoes rich in taste.

- 1 pound ripe, red tomatoes, chopped
- 3 spring onions or 1 small onion, diced
- 2 garlic cloves, chopped finely or minced
- 1/2 cucumber, peeled and diced
- 1/3 red bell pepper, diced
- 1/3 green or yellow bell pepper, diced
- 2 tablespoons olive oil
- 1 tablespoon sherry vinegar
- Salt and pepper

Place all ingredients in a blender and blend until smooth. Pass the soup through a fine sieve (strainer). Chill in the refrigerator before serving. Add salt and pepper to taste.

Roasted Beet Soup

- 1 pound medium beets
- 1 clove garlic, chopped finely or minced
- 1 small onion, diced
- 1 carrot, diced
- 1-2 tablespoon dill, finely chopped
- 2 tablespoons olive oil
- 3-4 cups chicken stock or vegetable stock
- 1 lemon
- Salt and pepper

Preheat oven to 350F. Roast the beets in parchment paper 1.5-2 hours, or until tender (you should be able to poke a skewer through the beets easily). Set aside to cool and then chop. Heat the oil on

Intermittent Blasting Recipes

medium-low heat in a heavy-based pan and add the onion and garlic. Cook gently for around 5-10 minutes, or until soft. Add the carrot and beet, stir in, and then add the stock. Simmer for around 45 minutes, or until the vegetables are soft. Serve or blend and serve, if you like. Squeeze the lemon, and add in the juice and the dill generously. Add salt and pepper, to taste.

Sweet Potato and Carrot Soup

- 1 small onion, diced
- 2 sweet potatoes, peeled and chopped (alternatively you can use butternut squash)
- 2 large carrots, diced
- 2 tablespoons extra-virgin olive oil
- 1 teaspoon ground cumin
- 1/2 teaspoon ground cardamom
- 1/2 teaspoon ground coriander seeds
- 2-4 cups organic chicken or vegetable stock

Heat the olive oil on medium/low heat in a heavy-based pan, add the onion, and cook on a low heat for a few minutes. Add the sweet potato, carrots and spices. Cook on low heat for 5-7 minutes, or until starting to soften, stirring occasionally. Add enough stock to cover the vegetables and simmer until they are soft. Put in the blender and blend until smooth.

Acorn Squash Soup

- 2 acorn squash
- Extra-virgin olive oil
- 2 shallots, chopped
- 1 good-sized white or yellow onion, diced finely
- Some aromatics of your choice, such as whole parsley or thyme sprigs, celery stems, and leaves, etc.
- Adobo blended with oregano and cumin, to taste
- Yellow curry powder, to taste (about 1-1/2 to 2 teaspoons)
- Salt, pepper, cumin

Intermittent Blasting Recipes

- 2 bay leaves
- 32 ounces of chicken or vegetable stock

Preheat oven to 350 degrees. Cut squash in half and scoop out seeds. Season with salt and pepper and roast, cut side up, for about an hour until toasty and soft. Cool. While squash is roasting and cooling, heat a Dutch oven over medium flame. Sauté onion and shallots in olive oil over medium to low heat. Season with adobo, curry, bay leaves, and peppers; throw in celery leaves/stems. Reduce heat a bit and let the mixture cook until caramelized a bit. Add stock. If you have some aromatics, such as thyme, flat-leaf parsley, etc. throw them into the stock mixture whole – you can easily fish them out when you're ready to finish the soup. When the stock mixture tastes right and squash is cooled, fish out any stems, bits of squash skin, bay leaves, etc., and scoop the squash flesh out of the skin, right into the stock mixture. Puree. Add salt, pepper, and cumin to taste and garnish with your favorite herbs.

Thai Sweet Potato and Carrot Soup

- 2-3 sweet potatoes or 1 butternut squash, diced
- 2-3 carrots, diced
- 1-2 tablespoons light olive oil
- 1 can coconut milk
- 1/2 organic chicken or vegetable stock cube
- 1 tablespoon red Thai curry paste
- 1 small knob ginger, finely chopped/minced
- 1 fat clove garlic, finely chopped or minced
- 1 bunch cilantro, finely chopped

Gently heat the oil in a heavy-based pan on medium to low heat and add the sweet potatoes or squash and carrots, ginger, and garlic, and sweat for 5-10 minutes or a little longer until they start to soften, stirring occasionally. Add the curry paste and stir in. Add the coconut milk, stock cube, and some water if required (depending on how thin or thick you want the soup to be). Simmer until the vegetables are soft, put in the blender, and serve with the cilantro.

Miso Soup with Noodles

- 1/2 cup uncooked noodles (e.g., buckwheat, wheat, or brown rice)
- 2 teaspoons sesame oil
- 1 small onion or shallot, chopped very fine
- 1 clove garlic, chopped or minced
- 2-3 cups water
- 1 tablespoon tamari sauce (if not gluten-sensitive, you can substitute soy sauce)
- 1 heaping tablespoon white miso paste (found in the refrigerated section of the grocery store)
- 1/2 cup broccoli, chopped
- 1/2 cup green beans, sliced
- Salt and pepper

Cook the noodles as directed. Take care not to overcook them or they will get overly soft when added to the hot soup. Heat sesame oil on medium heat in a heavy-based pan and add the onions. Cook for one minute, then add the garlic and cook for about 30 seconds. Add the water, tamari sauce, and miso paste and bring to a boil. Add the vegetables and cook for 2-3 minutes so they are still crunchy. Add the noodles and serve. Add additional tamari sauce, to taste, if necessary. Add salt and pepper, to taste.

Salads / Salad Dressings

Salads are quick to make, they are an excellent source of nutrients and fiber, and they are also very versatile. These recipes are intended as a guide and lend themselves to all kinds of variations – you can improvise according to what you enjoy, what's in season or what you happen to have in your kitchen. Eat them as a meal or as an accompaniment to other dishes – the aim of these salad ideas is

Intermittent Blasting Recipes

to help boost your intake of raw, delicious vegetables when transitioning from your Intermittent Blast. You can also enjoy them every day, but not while you are on your Intermittent Blast.

Simple Olive Oil and Lemon Dressing

- 3 tablespoons extra-virgin olive oil
- 1 tablespoon lemon juice
- 1/2 to 1 clove garlic, minced
- Salt and pepper, to taste
- 1/2 teaspoon honey (optional)

Stir or shake ingredients together until well-blended. This dressing goes well with most any salad. I usually just pour the olive oil and lemon juice on my salad and add salt, pepper and herbs to taste with or without garlic.

Olive Oil and Raw Apple-Cider Vinegar Dressing

Raw apple-cider vinegar has some remarkable health- promoting properties – it is antibacterial, it contains bone-and muscle-friendly calcium and magnesium, it strengthens immunity, it aids digestion, it alkalizes the body, it can relieve sore throats and sinus infections, it is a natural appetite-suppressant, and it can even relieve the symptoms of arthritis. It makes a delicious dressing that goes well with most salads.

- 3 tablespoons extra-virgin olive oil
- 1 tablespoon raw apple cider vinegar
- 1 teaspoon Dijon mustard
- 1 small garlic clove, chopped small or minced
- Salt and pepper, to taste

Shake ingredients together until well-blended and drizzle over salads, steamed vegetables, avocados or any other foods you enjoy.

Avocado Sesame Salad

- 1 avocado, sliced

Intermittent Blasting Recipes

- 1 carrot, sliced
- 1/2 cup fine green beans
- 1 cup salad leaves
- 1/2 cup arugula (rocket)
- 2 teaspoons sesame seeds

Dressing:

- 3 tablespoons extra-virgin olive oil
- 1 tablespoon balsamic vinegar
- 1 teaspoon mustard

Heat the sesame seeds in a dry pan on medium-low heat until they start to crack. Place the salad ingredients in a salad bowl. Mix the dressing by shaking the ingredients together in a jar with a lid until fully blended together. Toss the salad ingredients with the dressing and immediately mix in the hot sesame seeds so that they crackle and give off an aroma.

Mediterranean Salad

- 1/2-1 cup green beans, lightly steamed
- 1/2-1 cup broccoli, cut into florets (raw or very lightly steamed)
- Handful lettuce leaves – any high-quality, local, seasonal lettuce you prefer
- Handful arugula (rocket) leaves
- Handful pitted black olives, Kalamata or olives of choice
- 3-4 artichoke hearts, from a jar or marinated
- 1-2 tablespoons sun-dried tomatoes (optional)

Mix ingredients together in bowl and pour the dressing over the top. Toss the salad and serve.

Greek Salad

Capers are fermented and revered for their digestive benefits. They also add piquancy to the flavor of an ordinary Greek salad.

Intermittent Blasting Recipes

- 2 tablespoons extra-virgin olive oil
- 1 tablespoon white wine vinegar or raw apple cider vinegar
- 1-2 cloves garlic, chopped small or minced
- 2 fresh tomatoes, sliced
- 1/2 cucumber, sliced
- 1/2 onion, sliced thin
- 1/2 cup Kalamata olives
- 1 tablespoon chopped fresh parsley
- 1 teaspoon ground oregano
- 2 teaspoons capers
- Salt and freshly-ground black pepper, to taste

Mix the oil, vinegar, and garlic together to make a dressing. Mix together the other ingredients, toss with the dressing, and season to taste.

Tomato and Basil Salad

This is, of course, a Mediterranean classic. It's a great use for ripe red tomatoes grown on the vine. The tomatoes provide the antioxidant lycopene, which is thought to be one reason why Mediterranean men have low rates of prostate cancer.

- 4-5 large ripe tomatoes
- Handful fresh basil leaves, torn
- Extra-virgin olive oil or an olive-oil-based salad dressing
- Freshly-ground black pepper

Slice the tomatoes thinly and mix in a bowl with the basil leaves. Drizzle with olive oil or salad dressing and black pepper, to taste. This recipe also goes well with avocados and/or thinly-sliced onion.

Beet and Carrot Salad

An important rule of healthy cuisine is that the food should look colorful and appetizing. Combining the orange and purple of this salad with a green salad (such as the baby spinach, watercress and arugula) will make a very colorful, nutrient-rich dish and the two salads together will complement most savory dishes.

- 1-2 beets uncooked, peeled, and julienned or shredded
- 2 large carrots, washed or peeled and finely sliced/julienned
- 2 tablespoons cilantro (coriander), chopped small
- 2-3 tablespoons seeds (pumpkin seeds, sunflower seeds, etc.)

Mix together, dress, and serve with an olive-oil-based salad dressing.

Baby Spinach, Watercress, and Arugula Salad

Dark leafy greens such as these are full of nutrients like iron and folate and are full of taste with a bit of a kick.

- 1 cup arugula (rocket)
- 1 cup watercress
- 1 cup baby spinach

Simply mix the leaves together and serve with an olive-oil-based dressing – this salad goes well with apple-cider vinegar, lemon, or balsamic vinegar dressings.

Fennel, Artichoke, and Lentil Salad

- 1/2-1 head fennel, sliced
- 1/2 cup artichoke hearts
- 1/2-1 cup cooked or canned green lentils
- 1 shallot, very finely chopped

Mix the ingredients together with an olive-oil-based dressing.

Zucchini and Carrot Salad

- 2 zucchini
- 2 large carrots
- 1/2 tablespoon chopped dill
- Juice of 1/2-1 lemon
- 1-2 tablespoon extra-virgin olive oil

Intermittent Blasting Recipes

For this salad you can slice the vegetables thinly, grate them, peel them in ribbons, or julienne them. Simply mix together, add dressing, and serve.

Japanese Salad

The Okinawans love their radishes and colorful, beautifully-arranged salads. This recipe goes well with Japanese dishes as well as with the Okinawan staple, the sweet potato.

- 2 spring onions
- 5-6 radishes
- 1/4 cucumber, with seeds removed
- 1/2 cup snow peas
- 1-2 medium carrots
- 1 celery stalk

Thinly slice or dice the celery, carrots, cucumber, and radishes, or cut into round slices, if you prefer. Serve with the dressing of choice.

Cucumber and Wakame Salad

Seaweed is ultra-high in nutrients, and green, stringy wakame is popular in salads. This is just one of many variations on seaweed salad, which is a staple in Japan and Okinawa.

- 1 cucumber, sliced thin
- 2 ounces wakame seaweed, rehydrated in water
- 4 tablespoons rice vinegar
- 1-2 tablespoons sesame seeds, briefly roasted
- 1/2 teaspoon salt

Sprinkle the cucumber with salt and set aside until the cucumber yields its water, then squeeze to remove moisture and pat dry. Combine with the seaweed, sesame seeds, and rice vinegar.

Bean Sprout Salad

Bean sprouts are popular in the Longevity Hot Spots Okinawa, Bama, and Hunza. Sprouting beans raises their nutrient content and makes them more digestible; sprouts are a very useful superfood to keep at home as you can simply throw a handful into salads or stir-fries to up the nutrient content. They will also make you feel fuller for longer, due to their content of protein and fiber.

- 1 carrot, cut into juliennes
- 1/2 cucumber, cut into juliennes and with seeds removed
- 5-10 fine green beans, cut into juliennes
- 1-2 cups sprouts (alfalfa sprouts, mung bean sprouts, broccoli sprouts, etc.)
- 2 tablespoons chopped cilantro

Mix together and dress with your dressing of choice, or with just a squeeze of lemon and olive oil.

Summer Peach and Tomato Salad

- 1 large peach
- 1 large tomato
- Balsamic reduction for drizzling

Slice the tomatoes and peaches to a medium thickness. Arrange on a plate. Drizzle with the balsamic reduction and serve.

Greek Salad, Symi Style

- 2 tablespoons extra-virgin olive oil
- 1 tablespoon white wine vinegar or raw apple cider vinegar
- 1-2 cloves garlic, chopped fine or minced
- 2 fresh tomatoes, sliced
- 1/2 cucumber, sliced
- 1/2 onion, sliced thin
- 1/2 cup black olives
- 1 tablespoon chopped fresh parsley

Intermittent Blasting Recipes

- 1 teaspoon oregano
- 2 teaspoons capers or a few large capers with stalks
- Salt and freshly-ground black pepper
- 2-3 large fresh sardines (If you can't find fresh sardines, use canned sardines)

Mix the oil, vinegar, and garlic together to make a dressing. Mix together the other ingredients. Then lay the sardines over the top. Toss with the dressing and season to taste.

Tuna Nicoise Salad

- 1 can tuna, drained
- 4 free-range eggs, hard-boiled and cut into quarters
- 3-1/2 tablespoons capers, chopped very small
- 3-1/2 ounces gherkins, chopped very small
- 3 potatoes, boiled and diced
- 2 onions, sliced very thin
- 3 tomatoes, chopped
- 3-1/2 tablespoons Nicoise olives
- 5-6 anchovy fillets
- 1 green bell pepper, chopped
- 1 red bell pepper, chopped
- 1 small head lettuce

Mix together the ingredients, shredding the lettuce if you wish, and serve with olive oil and raw apple-cider vinegar dressing.

Quick Salad with Beans or Lentils

This makes a very useful, quick, inexpensive, filling, nutrient-rich lunch or supper and is especially convenient if you want to take something to the office or on the road. This also goes well with soup; if you are having an office lunch, try making soup in batches and freezing it, then heating it up in the morning and taking it with you in a food flask to accompany your salad.

Intermittent Blasting Recipes

- 1 can beans, or 2 cups beans which have been soaked overnight and cooked (borlotti beans, kidney beans, cannellini beans, black-eyed peas, black beans)
- 2 tablespoons fresh seeds (pumpkin or sunflower)
- 2 cups salad vegetables of your choice – carrot, cucumber, tomato, lettuce, fennel, celery, watercress, arugula
- Fresh herbs (optional)
- Olive-oil-based salad dressing

Simply mix ingredients and add dressing just before serving.

Transition Entrees

These entrees can be enjoyed on non-Intermittent Blasting days or while transitioning from your Intermittent Blast back to your normal diet. They are very nutritious and delicious!

Lentil Shepherd's Pie

This is a simple vegetarian version of ordinary shepherd's pie. If desired, you can cook other vegetables with the lentils, such as chopped zucchini, broccoli florets cut small, and/or chopped bell peppers.

- 14 ounces lentils (green or brown)
- 3-4 potatoes for mashing
- 1 tablespoon butter (optional – for the potatoes)
- 1 onion, chopped
- 2 cloves garlic, minced
- 1 carrot, chopped
- 1 stalk celery, finely chopped
- 2 tomatoes, chopped
- 1 heaping tablespoon tomato paste
- 1 tablespoon vegetable stock powder or 1 vegetable stock cube
- 2 tablespoons olive oil
- 1 teaspoon mixed herbs

- Freshly-ground black pepper

Scrub or peel the potatoes, cut them in half, and boil them in water until tender. Meanwhile, gently cook or sweat the onion, celery, carrot, and garlic in the olive oil in a pan for 5 minutes, or until the vegetables are softening. Add the vegetable stock with a splash of water and mix in. Add the tomato paste and cook for another 3-4 minutes. Stir in the lentils, herbs, and pepper to taste. Mash the potatoes and add butter. You can substitute olive oil for butter, if desired. Place the lentil mixture in a baking dish and layer the potatoes on top. Cook in the oven at 350 degrees for 40-50 minutes.

Salmon with Lentils

Salmon and lentils make a good culinary match and both are great sources of protein. You can try your own variations of this basic recipe. This dish goes well with a large salad or lightly-cooked green vegetables, such as spinach, watercress, zucchini, broccoli, asparagus, or green beans.

- 5 to 7 ounces salmon
- 1 can Puy lentils or 2 cups Puy lentils, soaked and cooked
- 1 onion, finely chopped
- 1 carrot, finely chopped
- 1 stalk celery, finely chopped
- 1 clove garlic, minced
- 1 bell pepper (any color), finely chopped
- 1/2 tablespoon vegetable bouillon powder, or 1/2 vegetable stock cube
- 1 tablespoon fresh dill, chopped
- Juice of 1 lemon
- Extra-virgin olive oil
- Salt and pepper

Preheat oven to 350 degrees. Place the salmon in an oven-safe dish, drizzle with olive oil, and season with salt, pepper, and herbs of choice, if desired. Cover with foil and cook in the oven for about 20-25 minutes, or until cooked through. Meanwhile, heat 1-2 tablespoons of olive oil in a heavy-based pan on medium heat and add the chopped vegetables. Cook, stirring, for 1-2 minutes. Add the vegetable bouillon powder or stock cube and a splash of water, and stir in. Cook for around 10 minutes on a medium-low heat until soft. Add the cooked or canned lentils and simmer gently for 5 minutes. Serve the lentils with the cooked salmon on top, sprinkled with lemon juice and the chopped dill.

Adzuki Bean Burgers

This is one of those recipes with which you can experiment with endless variations of your own. Try adding sun-dried tomatoes, chili pepper, mustard, or different herbs. Serve with a big green salad.

- 1 can adzuki beans or 2 cups adzuki beans, soaked overnight and cooked
- 1 cup millet or quinoa, cooked
- 1 red onion, finely chopped
- 1 stalk celery, finely chopped
- 1 carrot, finely chopped
- 1-2 cloves garlic, minced
- 1 tablespoon parsley or cilantro (coriander), finely chopped
- 2 tablespoons olive oil
- Salt and freshly-ground black pepper

Heat the olive oil in a heavy-based pan on medium-low heat and cook the red onion and garlic for 2-3 minutes. Then add the rest of the vegetables and cook for a another 5 minutes until soft. Remove from the heat and put the mixture into a food processor. Add the quinoa and adzuki beans and blend until they are well-combined. Add the parsley or cilantro, pepper to taste and a pinch of salt, if desired. Put the mixture in a bowl and refrigerate for 30-60 minutes. Remove and form into small patties. To do this, make a ball and then flatten it slightly between your palms. Place the burgers on a lightly-oiled baking tray and cook at 350 degrees for 30-35 minutes, turning the burgers over once mid-way through cooking.

Gallo Pinto (Costa Rican rice and beans)

Gallo pinto translates literally as 'spotted rooster' in Spanish; the origin of this Costa Rican classic is disputed, but one theory is that it was introduced to Latin America by Afro-Latino immigrants. Ask any Nicoyan what they have eaten that day, and they are bound to have had gallo pinto, quite likely for every meal (yes, including breakfast). This dish is best accompanied by a salad, guacamole, salsa, and/or a generous helping of vegetables.

- 2 tablespoons olive oil
- 1 onion, finely chopped
- 2 cloves garlic, minced
- A pinch of chili pepper (optional)
- 1 teaspoon ground cumin (optional)
- 1 teaspoon ground cilantro (coriander) seed (optional)
- 1 red bell pepper, finely chopped
- 2-3 cups cooked brown rice
- 2 cups cooked or canned black beans or kidney beans, liquid reserved
- 1 tablespoon cilantro (coriander), chopped
- Salt and pepper

Heat the oil on medium-low heat in a heavy-based pan. Add the onion and cook for 2-3 minutes. Then add the garlic and bell pepper. Add the ground cilantro and cumin seed at this stage, if you choose to use them. Cook gently or sweat for a another 5 minutes, or until the vegetables are soft. Add the beans and then the rice, as well as the chili pepper; heat through and season. Add a little of the bean liquid, if necessary. Serve with the cilantro.

Intermittent Blasting Recipes

Buckwheat Wraps

Buckwheat flour is useful for making wraps if you wish to avoid gluten – it folds over better than rice flour wraps (buckwheat is not technically a grain, but a seed, and may cause allergies in some people). Rye flour also works well and is a good substitute for wheat, but is not gluten-free.

- Buckwheat or rye flour (1/2 cup makes 2-3 wraps)
- Water
- Salt

Place the flour and a pinch of salt in a bowl and add a little water. Mix together with a fork and work into a paste. Add water and keep mixing until you have a fairly thin pancake-like mixture. Heat olive oil on medium heat in a heavy-based pan. Put the pancake mixture into the pan and cook until the wrap is starting to turn golden on each side and a little crispy around the edges.

Amy's Lemon-Rosemary Salmon

- 4 (6-ounce) salmon fillets
- 1/4 cup extra-virgin olive oil
- 1 tablespoon minced fresh rosemary
- 8 lemon slices
- 1/4 cup lemon juice
- 1/2 cup white wine
- 4 teaspoons capers
- 4 pieces of natural parchment paper
- Salt and freshly ground black pepper, to taste

Preheat oven to 350°. Rub top and bottom of salmon fillets with olive oil. Season with salt, pepper, and rosemary. Place a piece of seasoned fish in the center of a piece of parchment paper. Top each piece of salmon with 2 lemon slices, 1 tablespoon of lemon juice, 2 tablespoons of wine, and 1 teaspoon of capers. Gather the ends of the paper together, fold down tightly and tuck the sides underneath. Repeat with remaining fish. Place in a shallow roasting pan and bake for 15-20 minutes. Serve with fresh, colorful vegetables, tomato chutney, and roasted potatoes.

Chapter 5: Healthy Eating Every Day!

Yes, I know I always say that when you Blast Intermittently, you can eat normally most of the time and still receive great health benefits, and, in fact, you can. Regardless of your "normal" diet, introducing a regimen of Intermittent Blasting will certainly help you get healthier, have more energy, and lose weight. However, if your "normal" diet consists of pizza and cheeseburgers, we need to talk.

If you couldn't tell by now, I've made health and nutrition my life's work. And I would be remiss if I did not touch upon some of the ideas and concepts that will help you enjoy a variety of healthy, nutritionally-dense recipes for you to sample when you are not Intermittent Blasting. The choice is yours. The Intermittent Blast will help you no matter what you eat when you are not Intermittent Blasting. But if you want to "fast-track" your way to optimal health, keep reading.

Snacks

Everyone loves to snack. In part, we were designed this way. The concept of "three meals a day" is pretty recent and until then, humans ate what they could, when they could, no matter how large or small the amount of food. Hence, "snacking" became incorporated into our DNA. But there is a big difference in today's world and it does make a difference if you snack on a candy bar or one of these delicious, nutritious options below.

Most of these snacks contain protein and beneficial fats, and you can also eat a piece of fruit or have a smoothie, which will sustain you very well. Don't feel that by having a snack you are adding calories and are therefore likely to gain weight. As long as you are hungry when you have the snack, just the opposite is true. Having a nutrient-rich snack will help keep your blood-sugar level even, which is key to maintaining your desired weight. Beneficial fats help steady your blood sugar and boost the metabolism, so don't be afraid of them. The main principle is that your snack should be modest in size and rich in nutrients (nutrient-dense). Sugary foods such as donuts, bagels or pastries are not good snacks to have because they are devoid of nutrients, increase blood sugar and are likely to lead to sugar cravings and weight gain. Try some of these:

- Fruit-and-vegetable smoothie
- Handful of nuts and seeds (raw is best)
- Handful of dried fruit and nuts
- Oatcakes with hummus
- Cut vegetables like celery, bell peppers, cucumbers, radishes with hummus
- Oat cakes with avocado and basil
- Carrots dipped in nut butter (sugar-free and without hydrogenated vegetable fats)
- Brown rice cakes with hummus and avocado or nut butter and fruit spread
- Smoothie with added soaked flax or chia seeds
- Piece of fruit
- Bowl of mixed berries (strawberries, blueberries, raspberries)
- Cut pieces of carrot, celery, cucumber, cauliflower, red pepper, broccoli, or any other raw vegetables, serve with healthy dips or dressings of choice

If you feel hungry during the day and need something to get you through to mealtime, these are healthy suggestions to keep you going. Otherwise you'll get too hungry, and may be in danger of getting a sugar or carb craving; it's just downhill from there.

Guacamole

Guacamole is a favorite in Costa Rica and regularly has its place on the side of the plate. Avocados are high in beneficial

Intermittent Blasting Recipes

monounsaturated fatty acids and heart-friendly vitamin E, while the other ingredients in guacamole provide a range of antioxidants and other nutrients. It's delicious with salad, bean dishes, in a sandwich or pita, or as a dip; raw carrots or celery go particularly well with it.

- 1-2 tablespoons cilantro, finely chopped
- 1 tomato, finely chopped
- 1 small onion, finely chopped
- The juice of one lime (use a lemon if you have no limes)
- 1-2 large avocados, mashed
- 1 small chili pepper, finely chopped
- Salt to taste

You can either mix the ingredients together as they are or you can first pound the onion, cilantro, chili pepper, tomato and salt into a paste before mixing with the avocado and lime juice. The guacamole should be a little chunky, so if you use a blender to mash the avocado, go easy. Eat soon after making – if you have any guacamole left over, keep the avocado seed in the mixture as it helps prevent it from going brown.

Salsa

Having salsa as an accompaniment to your dishes will add not only an exciting bit of flavor, but also some powerful health benefits. The tomatoes provide the antioxidant lycopene, the onions and garlic are immune-boosting, the chili peppers contain anti-inflammatory, antibacterial capsaicin, the lime provides vitamin C, and the cilantro is extra-high in antioxidants. It is also low in calories, but will boost the feeling of satiety, due to its high nutrient content.

- 1-2 cloves garlic, peeled and finely chopped or minced
- 1 onion, finely chopped
- 3 large ripe tomatoes, finely chopped
- 1-2 chili peppers, finely chopped
- 3 tablespoons cilantro, finely chopped
- The juice of one lime

Intermittent Blasting Recipes

- Salt and pepper to taste

Simply combine the ingredients in a bowl. If the mixture seems too dry, you can add a tablespoonful of water. Refrigerate for 2-4 hours to combine. Serve with Mexican dishes, tapas, as a dip, with guacamole, or any way you like.

Traditional Hummus

- 1 (15 ounce) can garbanzo beans (chickpeas), drained
- 3 tablespoons olive oil
- 1 tablespoon lemon juice
- 3 tablespoons tahini
- 4 cloves garlic, minced
- 1/4 cup water
- 1 pinch paprika

Mix garbanzo beans, 2 tablespoons olive oil, tahini, lemon juice, water, and garlic, in a food processor or blender until smooth. Transfer to a bowl. Drizzle 1 tablespoon olive oil over it and sprinkle paprika on top.

Dairy-Free Pesto

- 2 cups basil leaves tightly packed
- 1/8 cup extra-virgin olive oil
- 1-2 teaspoon crushed garlic
- Salt to taste
- 1/8 cup raw pine nuts or raw almond slivers (chopped finely)

Chop all ingredients in a food processor until well blended. Great with meats and seafood.

Chunky Sweet Potato Salsa

- 3 medium sweet potatoes, peeled and chopped into small cubes
- 1 red pepper, chopped
- 1 large avocado, diced

Intermittent Blasting Recipes

- 1 large shallot, sliced
- 1 cup blackberries
- 1/2 cup cilantro, chopped
- 1 tablespoon extra-virgin olive oil
- 1/2 teaspoon cinnamon
- 1/4 teaspoon nutmeg
- 1/2 teaspoon raw honey
- 1 teaspoon fresh lime juice
- 1/2 teaspoon raw apple-cider vinegar
- Salt and pepper

Preheat oven to 350 degrees. Keeping each ingredient separate, chop the red pepper, avocado, cilantro and shallots. In a medium bowl, combine the sweet potatoes, olive oil, cinnamon, nutmeg, salt and pepper. Stir until sweet potatoes are coated. Line a baking sheet with parchment paper and pour the sweet potatoes onto the sheet. Bake for 10-12 minutes. Turn the sweet potatoes over and add the sliced shallots. Bake for another 20-25 minutes. In a small bowl, whisk together the honey, lime juice, vinegar, and salt and pepper. After the sweet potatoes and shallots have baked, put them in a large bowl and add the red pepper, avocado, blackberries, and cilantro. Pour the dressing over the top of the vegetable mixture and fold until coated. Serve with organic corn chips or cut vegetables.

Dahl with Lemon and Coriander

Dahl (lentils) provide fiber to keep the intestines healthy and protein for sustained energy.

- 1 can drained lentils or two cups cooked lentils (brown, black or yellow)
- 1 large onion, shredded
- 2 tablespoons extra-virgin olive oil, ghee, or clarified butter

Intermittent Blasting Recipes

- 3 tomatoes, finely chopped
- 2 tablespoons tomato paste
- 2-3 fresh green chili peppers, finely chopped
- 2 teaspoons garam masala or curry powder
- The juice of 2 lemons
- 1 bunch cilantro (coriander), chopped
- Salt to taste
- Water

Wash lentils well and place in pan with 17 fluid ounces of water. Bring to a boil and cook (how long this takes depends on the type of lentils; it may be as little as 15-20 minutes or could be longer). In the meantime, heat the oil on medium-low heat in a heavy-based pan, add the onion, and cook for 3-5 minutes until soft. Add the tomatoes, tomato paste, and chilies and cook for around 5 minutes, stirring occasionally. Add the garam masala or curry powder and a little salt to taste, if desired. When the lentils are cooked, add them to the mixture and simmer for 5 minutes. Add extra tomato paste and/or water if the dhal is too dry. Squeeze in the lemon juice and coriander and serve.

Healthy Treats

We all like to indulge our sweet-tooth every once in a while. That's a perfectly normal desire. But why reach for candy or sugar-coated sweets when there are delicious options that are both sweet and nutritious? Here are some great treats that help curb our cravings for sweets.

No-Bake Fudge Brownies

- Coconut oil
- 4 1/2 cups pecans
- 3/4 cup pitted dates, packed
- 3/4 cup raw cacao powder
- 1/4 teaspoon ground cinnamon

- 1 teaspoon maca powder
- 1 teaspoon ground vanilla powder
- 1/2 teaspoon salt
- 1/4 teaspoon cayenne pepper (optional)
- 1/4 cup dried black cherries, goji berries, golden berries, or mulberries
- 1/4 cup hemp seeds, reserved

Grease an 8x8 inch glass baking dish with coconut oil. In a food processor, process the pecans until slightly chunky (do not over-process into pecan butter). Place 1/2 cup pecans in a separate bowl and set aside. While food processor is running, slowly add dates, rocking base of food processor to combine evenly. Add cacao, cinnamon, maca, vanilla, salt, and cayenne and process again until well-combined. Fold in dried fruit, hemp seeds, and remaining pecans. Spread mixture into baking dish, pressing down with your palms. Refrigerate for 30 minutes to set, then cut into squares. Makes 10 bars.

Go Green Ice Pops

- 3 medium bananas
- 2 cups fresh pineapple chunks
- 2 cups fresh spinach
- 1 cup water, milk of choice (coconut, almond, hemp), or 100% natural pineapple juice (depending on creaminess or sweetness desired)

Blend spinach and liquid of choice. Add pineapple and purée. Add bananas and continue to blend until you have a smoothie-like consistency. Pour in popsicle molds and freeze (typically takes 1 to 3 hours).

Strawberry Basil Ice Pops

- 2 cups strawberries
- 3 tablespoons honey

- 2 tablespoons lemon juice
- 2 tablespoons basil leaves, chopped

Purée the strawberries with the honey, lemon juice, and basil leaves. Pour in molds and freeze.

Banana Oatmeal Raisin Cookies

- 3 ripe bananas, mashed
- 1/3 cup applesauce
- 2 cups oats
- 1/4 cup almond milk
- 1/4 cup raisins
- 1 teaspoon vanilla
- 1 teaspoon cinnamon

Mix all ingredients and bake at 350 degrees for 15-20 minutes.

Three-Berry Chia Pudding

- 2 cups unsweetened almond or coconut milk
- 1-1/2 cups fresh blueberries, blackberries and raspberries
- 2 tablespoons chia seeds
- 1/8 teaspoon raw honey

Combine the milk together with the chia seeds and fruit in a glass jar with a lid. Cover and shake well; set aside for 15 minutes. Give it another good shake, and then refrigerate overnight or at least 5-6 hours. Divide into 2 bowls or glass serving dishes and serve.

No-Bake Cinnamon Apple Dessert

- 6 apples
- 3 cups water
- 3 tablespoons cinnamon
- 3 tablespoons vanilla extract
- 3 tablespoons sugar or healthy substitute
- Juice from one lemon

Intermittent Blasting Recipes

Peel and core apples and cut them into chunks. Toss everything except water together in a large pot. Apply heat until you hear the apples start to sizzle, and then add water. Cook until apples are thick and soft. You can cook on medium-low heat for 30-40 minutes, or on low heat for a couple of hours if you would like to keep the apples as chunks. Cook apples until soft and remove from liquid. Add cooked apples and serve.

Chapter 6: Superfoods

The Amazing Power of Superfoods

Whether you are Intermittent Blasting or not, always, always, always think about Blasting your body with nutrition at every opportunity. The way to do this is by constantly consuming Superfoods.

To perform optimally and to look and feel your best, your body requires quality nutrition and lots of it. It is estimated that up to 95% of Americans are deficient in the nutritional minerals that are essential for health. Most of us are running a nutritional deficient and this must change if we are to look and feel our best and maintain a healthy body weight, not to mention protect ourselves from sickness and disease. The way to accomplish this is by blasting your body with nutritional superfoods all the time.

What Exactly Are Superfoods?

These are the most nutritious, nutrient-dense foods on the planet. Pound for pound, ounce for ounce these foods provide the most bang for the buck when it comes to getting nutrition to your cells. These foods should be consumed at every opportunity. Oh, and most of them are delicious! Here are some examples of superfoods and the benefits they provide.

Acai Berries

The acai (ah-sah-ee) fruit is a small purple berry grown in Brazil, where it is commonly consumed by the locals. The Acai berry has become well known of late and deservedly so. This is a true superfood. It has an extremely high rating on the ORAC (oxygen radical absorbance capacity) score, which is a measure of antioxidant power. Eating a handful of acai berries daily will provide a powerful anti-aging effect. Acai also contains anthocyanins, fiber, plant sterols, and both omega 6 and omega 3 essential fatty acids, which is rare for a fruit. Acai contains about five hundred times more vitamin C than oranges.

How to eat: Acai berries are sold freeze-dried or can be found in supplements. Add a handful to your smoothies, crepes, or yogurt.

Remember: There is a delicate balance of free radicals and antioxidant levels in our bodies that needs to be maintained, since free radicals do not exist without reason and they do have their uses. Super-dosing acai supplements (and other antioxidant supplements) is not advisable. Acai berries are best used in their whole fruit form in moderation as part of a balanced diet.

Apples

It might not be exotic or flashy, but don't forget the humble apple! Apples contain antioxidant vitamins and are also one of the best sources of pectin, a soluble fiber that helps keep blood cholesterol levels low, blood glucose levels steady, and toxic heavy metals where they should be—out of your digestive tract. Apples also provide insoluble fiber, which helps sweep the intestines clean.

How to eat: Slice and add to fruit salad, smoothies, or desserts. Gently stew and puree them, or simply eat them as they are. Chewing the seeds will also provide you with vitamin B17, which might have the ability to kill cancer cells. Buy organic, locally-grown apples in season, if you can, and eat while fresh.

Apricots

Apricots became known as an important anti-aging food in the 1970s when Westerners discovered apricot trees dotted all over the Hunza valley, home to the legendary long-lived Hunzakuts of Pakistan. The bright orange fruit is spread out over the roofs of the houses to dry after harvesting and eaten in large quantities all year long.

Apricots are a rich source of minerals, fiber, and antioxidant beta carotene, especially when dried. Hunzakuts also crack open and eat the almond-like apricot kernels, which contain protein and omega 6 essential fatty acid. The kernels are also the best-known source of anti-cancer vitamin B17.

How to use: Eat dried or fresh on their own, together with a handful of kernels or almonds as an energy-boosting snack. Or eat as jam, or added to oat bars, or desserts.

Avocados

Avocados were once known by the Aztecs as "the fertility fruit." Today we know just how life-giving avocados can be. They're full of...

- Immune-enhancing plant sterols
- Protein
- Fiber
- The powerful antioxidant glutathione
- The antioxidant lutein
- Fat-soluble vitamin E, which protects cell membranes and blood vessels
- Fructo-oligo-saccharides, the fibers that encourage friendly bacteria to flourish in our intestines.

In addition, avocados contain monounsaturated fat, a healthy fat that can lower LDL cholesterol levels. This fat also aids absorption of fat-soluble vitamins; one study found that eating them with tomatoes and/or carrots raises absorption of prostate-protecting lycopene by up to 4.5 times and anti-cancer beta-carotene by 13.6 times (4). Avocados also contain their own carotenoids and have been found to inhibit the growth of prostate cancer cells in vitro (5). They are high in potassium, making them useful for lowering water retention.

How to eat: Cut avocados in half and eat with salad dressing. Add to salads or mix with pumpkin seeds, add to sandwiches, or as guacamole. Believe it or not, avocado makes a delicious addition to a fruit-and-vegetable smoothie.

Especially good lycopene and beta-carotene-boosting combinations are avocado with salsa; avocado with tomato, mozzarella and basil; and avocado with carrot, cottage cheese, and basil in a sandwich. Avocado oil, a rich source of vitamin E and monounsaturated fats, can be used to make salad dressings and can be used for cooking at high heat as it has a high smoke point.

Blueberries

Blueberries, as indicated by their rich color, are particularly high in the prized antioxidants anthocyanin and proanthocyanidin. They also rank high on the ORAC antioxidant score for fruits, with 2,234 units per 100g. Proanthocyanidins have the unusual ability to pass through the blood-brain barrier to enter the brain, where they can protect nerve tissue, help form new pathways, and help regenerate brain cells. Studies on rats have shown that blueberry consumption can actually reverse cognitive decline (6).

Proanthocyanidins do more good things:

- Improve circulation
- Reduce inflammation
- Protect blood vessels
- Neutralize free radicals

They've also been shown to be twenty times more effective than vitamin C and fifty times more effective than vitamin E in preventing oxidant damage, which is linked to accelerated aging. They greatly enhance the action of vitamin C, which is why sailors in the sixteenth century were saved from scurvy by eating lemons along with proanthocyanidin-rich pine bark.

Other red, blue, and purple berries—strawberries, cranberries, raspberries, and blackberries—are also high in anthocyanins and

Intermittent Blasting Recipes

proanthocyanidins and are an excellent anti-aging food. Most, including blueberries, also contain ellagic acid, a compound which causes cancer cells to self-destruct in a process called apoptosis.

How to eat: When in season, have a bowlful of blueberries and other berries daily and always use them in smoothies. You can also make homemade ice cream or frozen yogurt with berries.

If you can find them, wild blueberries have up to 100 times the amount of antioxidants as cultivated ones and are also relatively high in omega 3 essential fats. A recent study showed that freezing blueberries enhances the nutrition, so check the frozen fruits section in your supermarket.

Beans

Beans are a quick, easy way to make a meal more filling and raise protein levels and are a healthy way to consume non-animal protein. Black beans, green beans, aduki beans, soy beans, fagioli beans, cannellini beans, lima beans, mung beans... they can all be found at your local grocery waiting for you to add them to soups, casseroles, and salads.

Beans are also plentiful in soluble and insoluble fiber, antioxidant flavonoids, phytosterols, minerals, and energy-boosting, heart-friendly B vitamins. Many beans also contain phytoestrogens, such as genistein, which are thought to protect against hormone-related cancers.

A study by Tulane University School of Public Health in New Orleans found that people who included beans in their diets at least four times a week lowered their heart disease risk by 22 percent, as compared to people whose diets included a serving or less each week.

How to eat: Add beans to onion, garlic, and tomatoes cooked in olive oil or grapeseed oil and add a spoonful of turmeric for a superfood quintuple-whammy. Then mash them up, sprinkle coriander and a little lemon juice over them, and serve in a buckwheat pancake.

You can also add them to casseroles and soups for a hearty and non-fattening meal. Or add beans to a salad for a quick, satisfying lunch. Sprouting beans prevents them from causing gas.

Brassica Vegetables

Brassica, or cruciferous, vegetables—like broccoli, cauliflower, cabbage, Brussels sprouts, bok choy, kale, and watercress—are what everyone should be eating if they want to lower the risk of cancer.

Epidemiological studies reveal a link between brassica-eating populations and lower cancer rates. In addition, brassicas have been shown in studies to prevent tumors in animals given a potent carcinogen or even exposed to radiation. They are eaten in plentiful quantities by the long-lived Okinawans, Sardinians, Campodimelani, and Hunzakuts.

Their cancer-preventive effect is likely due to a range of compounds working together, almost as if they were designed to do so just for our benefit. Sulforaphane and indole-3-carbinol help the liver eliminate carcinogens during detoxification.

Vitamin C, calcium, magnesium, folic acid, selenium, carotenoids, and fiber have a synergistic antioxidant, anti-inflammatory, immune-boosting, and toxin-neutralizing effect. Brassicas also increase levels of an enzyme which converts estradiol into a safer form, thus possibly protecting against hormonal cancers such as breast cancer.

How to eat: Steam or lightly stir-fry brassicas, as cooking degrades the beneficial chemicals. They also taste better when they are crunchier. Cut small and add raw to salads, or use as dips. One study showed that just one or two servings of raw broccoli per month significantly reduced bladder cancer risk.

Intermittent Blasting Recipes

Buckwheat

Buckwheat is highly digestible, nutrient-rich, gluten-free—and, in spite of its name, has no relation to wheat. Buckwheat flour, used for baking and making noodles, comes from the seed of the plant.

Buckwheat bread is given to the Hunzakuts when they are ill, while the Japanese can be found downing buckwheat noodles when they have a hangover. Buckwheat's many beneficial properties include:

- Rutin, which supports capillary health
- Anti-cancer vitamin B-17
- Protein, fiber, and minerals such as iron, zinc, and selenium
- A protein that is thought to bind to cholesterol, thus lowering LDL cholesterol levels
- A compound, called D-chiro-inositol, which is involved in insulin use and is being studied for use in treating Type II diabetes
- Buckwheat also contains choline, a B vitamin that supports liver health—hence the hangover cure.

How to eat: Make pancakes easily and quickly by combining buckwheat and water with a little salt, then frying in olive or coconut oil. Make the mixture fairly runny. Spread in a thin layer and cook until golden. Serve with smoked salmon, dill, chopped spring onion, and crème fraiche. You can also make versatile breakfast pancakes with buckwheat by adding egg, vanilla, oat milk, and/or bananas and raisins. Buckwheat noodles are also available from Asian stores and health-food outlets and are good with mushrooms, soy sauce, garlic, and sesame oil.

Chocolate (cacao)

Cacao nibs, from which modern chocolate is derived, have a long history of medicinal use. Perhaps surprisingly, they rate near the top of the ORAC score for antioxidant levels (28,000 units per 100g). That's higher than any fruit or vegetable!

Dark chocolate has been found to lower heart disease risk by 20 percent, probably because it can:

- Reduce total cholesterol
- Reduce blood clots and inflammation in arteries
- Keep arteries elastic

There are still more unexpected benefits to cacao and chocolate. They are:

- Vasodilators, meaning they can lower blood pressure.
- High in magnesium, required by women during menstruation. That might be why women sometimes crave chocolate before their menstrual period.
- Sources of theobromine, which increases feelings of well-being, and phenylethylamine, a chemical released when we are in love.

One study, called the "sweet babies" study, found that mothers who ate chocolate while pregnant had happier children (11).

How to eat: Choose chocolate that is at least 70 percent cocoa. Eat it in small amounts since chocolate also contains sugar. Cacao is also available as a nutritional supplement.

Chlorella and Spirulina

These ancient species of algae have developed a reputation for having miraculous healing powers—and not without reason. Much-studied by scientists, they are extremely nutrient-dense and have been found to possess antiviral, anti-tumor, antibacterial, and anti-HIV properties.

They induce apoptosis (cell "suicide") in diseased liver cells and decrease blood pressure in hypertensive rats (12, 13). These important superfoods are even being hailed as the answer to some of the planet's 21st-century problems of nutrient deficiency.

Spirulina is a blue-green algae containing around 100 nutrients and a very high protein content of 60 to 70 percent. This superfood:

- Contains all eight essential amino acids that we need, making it a complete protein.
- Is rich in the antioxidants lutein, alpha-carotene, and beta-carotene.
- Contains remarkably high levels of gamma-linolenic acid (GLA).

Spirulina has also been found in studies to reduce viral replication, including HIV-1, mumps, and measles.

Chlorella is a green algae with 58% protein content and the complete set of essential amino acids. This superfood is:

- One of the few vegan sources of bioavailable vitamin B12.
- A rich source of chlorophyll, which can chelate toxins from the body and cleanse the bowel, liver, and bloodstream
- The source of chlorella growth factor, which has the potential to repair human genetic material and therefore has significant anti-aging powers.

Both algae contain a wide range of the minerals and trace elements our bodies need, as well as vitamins, essential fatty acids, antioxidants, and phytochemicals. They are also high in calcium and magnesium, which work together to improve our bone density. They are also thought to have prebiotic compounds to which support growth of the friendly intestinal flora you need to be healthy.

All of these benefits add up to a super-superfood with the potential to detoxify the body, improve immunity, rebuild nerve tissue, improve mental function, aid in bone health, and help prevent or even reverse disease.

How to use: Spirulina and chlorella are available as a powder, capsule, or tablet, both together and separately. Purchase from a reputable company and take as directed.

Cinnamon

As with all spices, cinnamon has antibacterial and anti-inflammatory qualities and is high in antioxidants. In fact, it measures almost off the scale on the ORAC score at 6,000 units per third of a teaspoon.

Cinnamon is a traditional remedy for flatulence, diarrhea, and other digestive problems. It's said that King Solomon took cinnamon as a remedy for his indigestion. Because of its chromium content, this spice may also have the potential to treat Type 2 diabetes.

How to use: Cinnamon comes as a stick or a powder. Dust it on your toast, pancakes, or soup. Drink as an herbal tea-make a tea with dried powdered bark or mix into ground coffee for cinnamon-flavored coffee. Cinnamon is also available as a supplement.

Caution: Because cinnamon has extremely high antioxidant levels, half a teaspoon is probably more than enough. Consuming high levels of antioxidants is not advisable—in fact, eating more than four tablespoons has been found to cause serious side-effects.

Flax

Flax seeds, an old favorite of Hippocrates, have earned their status as a superfood due to their high content of plant lignans, sterols, isoflavones, omega 3 fatty acids, protein, and fiber. Flax is the best source of plant lignans, which have the power to redirect estrogen metabolism and thus might help prevent hormone-related cancers of the breast, endometrium, and ovaries (14), (15). (The next best source? Sesame seeds.)

Flax is also rich in phytosterols, cholesterol-like plant fats that have been shown to lower LDL cholesterol levels in men and women

(16), (17). Exciting new research suggests that phytosterols are immune-modulating and therefore may be a valid treatment for autoimmune diseases such as multiple sclerosis and other diseases of the immune system, including HIV. Several studies also suggest that sterols may reduce the risk of cancers of the breast and prostate, stomach, lung, and endometrium, although it is not known whether this is due to the sterols in flax alone (18-21).

Early human diets were rich in phytosterols. But now they're lacking, partly because of farming methods and partly because of our diet. Eating flax is a good way to raise your phytosterol levels to where they should be. Nuts and seeds generally are an excellent source of protein, sterols, minerals, fiber, and essential fats.

How to use: Mix ground flax with applesauce, in yogurt, or in smoothies. You can cook with flax without destroying the lignans, so you can use it in baking. Buy the seeds, grind enough for three days, and keep the seeds in an airtight jar in the fridge. Or, buy from a dark-vacuum packet and store in the fridge.

You can also soak the seeds overnight and drink the gel-like mixture in the morning, or add it to a smoothie. This is excellent for cleaning the colon.

Garlic

Garlic—once known as the stinking rose—has a long tradition as a cure-all. It was used medicinally by Hippocrates as well as by monks in the Middle Ages to ward off the Plague.

Garlic has a long list of healing qualities:

- Protects against gastric and colorectal cancer
- Boosts immunity
- Lowers blood pressure and cholesterol
- Prevents colds

Intermittent Blasting Recipes

It has antibacterial, antiviral, antifungal, and anti-inflammatory properties—to the extent that it was used by the Russian army during World War II to keep wounds clean. As an antifungal, it is a useful treatment for candida, especially as it does not kill friendly bacteria. Garlic and onions are both good sources of quercetin, an effective natural antihistamine.

Garlic can protect against cancer in several ways:

- Kills H. pylori, the bacterium linked with stomach cancer.
- Is one of the best sources of organosulfur compounds, which have been found to slow the growth of prostate cancer cells in vitro.
- Contains the mineral selenium, which is linked to low cancer rates.

A meta-analysis of studies on garlic and cancer found that those with the highest garlic intakes had a 50 percent lower risk of gastric cancer than those with low intake and a 30 percent lower risk of colorectal cancer (22).

How to use: Crush or mince and use raw in salad dressings and dips, such as tzatziki. Lightly sweat garlic as a base for cooked dishes such as stews and soups, just as the Symiots, Campodimelani, Sardinians, and Hunzakuts (all Longevity Hot Spots) do.

Cooking garlic destroys some of the beneficial enzymes and cooked garlic has been found in studies to lose its cancer-protective qualities (23). However, letting the garlic stand for ten minutes after chopping and before heating preserves some of the active enzymes. Eat the real thing! Research shows that garlic itself is more useful than garlic supplements, which can vary in quality.

Ginger

Ginger is well-known for relieving nausea during pregnancy and after surgery, as well as for being a remedy for coughs and colds. It is anti-inflammatory, antiviral, and antioxidant.

Ginger also contains pungent antioxidant compounds, gingerol and zingerone, which may protect against heart disease and cancer. Gingerol relaxes blood vessels, thins the blood, and stimulates blood flow thus protecting heart health and boosting circulation. It has also been found to prevent the development of tumors in animals. Zingerone has been found to reduce damage to cells in mice that have been exposed to radiation (24, 25).

How to use: Drink as herb tea, juice for a quick shot, or simply add to your favorite fresh juice. Add freshly chopped ginger to marinades and stir-fries. Try it pickled with sushi, or dried and powdered in baking.

Goji Berries

These tangy, red, raisin-like berries have a long history of use in Chinese medicine. They rate up there with acai berries on the ORAC scale at 25,300 units—meaning you need just 20 grams (less than a handful) to reach your daily recommended intake of antioxidants.

Goji berries also contain high levels of phytochemicals—including 33 minerals and trace minerals, amino acids, vitamins, essential fatty acids, phytosterols, and carotenoids. Working together, these nutrients are likely to protect against chronic degenerative disease, including heart disease and cancer.

One of the carotenoids found in goji berries is zeaxanthin, which helps protect the retina of the eye from UV damage. Goji berries might help prevent age-related macular degeneration.

How to use: Goji berries usually come in dried form. They can be eaten raw or brewed into a tea.

Caution: It's not advisable to drink goji berries in a concentrated liquid form if you take blood-thinning drugs.

Green Tea

Green tea first had its moment when epidemiologists noticed that Japanese green-tea workers in one particular area seemed to have extremely low incidence of cancer.

It's now been shown that drinking several cups of strong green tea per day can help prevent cancer—particularly cancers of the breast, colon, prostate, lung, skin, bladder, stomach, and esophagus. The key substance is probably an antioxidant called epigallocatechin-3-gallate (EGCG), which has been found to kill cancer cells in human tissue and to prevent tumor growth in mice (26, 27).

Green tea also:

- Contains B vitamins for energy and immunity.
- Has more vitamin C than an orange.
- Contains vitamin E, which protects heart health by keeping the blood from coagulating.
- Protects against the inflammation that's linked to aging diseases like osteoporosis and heart disease.

Drinking green and black tea has been found in studies to lower levels of C-reactive protein, a marker of inflammation closely linked to heart disease.

Green tea can help you lose excess weight by improving insulin use so that glucose is burned for energy rather than being stored as fat; it also enhances fat-burning enzymes in cells. Furthermore, scientists have found that these two effects work together in a way that equals much more than the sum of their parts.

Green tea offers other benefits, such as:

- Antibacterial and antiviral properties.
- A prebiotic effect, meaning that it creates the right environment in the gut for friendly flora.

EGCG and other catechins are excellent for liver health and detoxification since they slow down the first phase of liver detoxification and enhance the second phase—enabling the dangerous intermediate chemicals formed after the first phase to be mopped up and eliminated more effectively.

People who are exposed to pollutants (almost everyone) tend to have an overly fast first phase of liver detoxification. So, drinking green tea can be very beneficial in this process since it gets rid of potential carcinogens.

How to use: Numerous studies have shown that the anti-cancer benefits are only noticeable in populations that consume four or more cups daily. The best-tasting green tea is made from leaves rather than teabags. It tastes especially good with lemongrass. The Okinawans have theirs scented with jasmine flowers—good health food shops often stock green tea with jasmine added.

Black tea, which is made from charred green tea leaves, also has health benefits. But the benefits are weaker, while the caffeine content is higher.

Mushrooms

Three types of mushrooms qualify for superfood status: maitake, shiitake, and reishi mushrooms.

Maitake is a Japanese word meaning "dancing mushroom," since Japanese mushroom hunters would traditionally dance for joy at finding one of these prized specimens. Maitake mushrooms:

- Contain compounds called beta-glucans, which have a powerful ability to strengthen our immune systems and are

known to increase levels of our tumor-fighting natural killer cells that suppress the growth of tumors (29).
- Contain X-fraction, which increases insulin sensitivity to help maintain a healthy weight and lower the risk of diabetes.
- Can lower blood pressure and blood lipids, which is why Japanese doctors use Maitake mushrooms to help protect against heart disease.

Shiitake mushrooms, which are eaten by the Okinawans, are high in anticancer vitamin D and a substance called lentinan that boosts immunity. Lentinan is used in Japan as an anti-tumor medicine.

The **reishi** mushroom, known in China as the plant of immortality, also has immune-boosting properties and is thought to protect heart health. Reishi is also used to treat asthma, respiratory conditions, liver disorders, and arthritis. It is anti-allergic, anti-inflammatory, antiviral, antibacterial, and antioxidant.

How to eat: Use in stir-fries, noodle dishes, soups, and other Asian dishes with garlic, sesame oil, and soy sauce. These mushrooms are also available in capsule form.

Spinach

Spinach is a common and powerful superfood. It is:

- Rich in protein
- High in minerals, including bone-friendly calcium and magnesium
- A good source of anti-aging alpha-lipoic-acid
- Rich in folic acid
- Full of vitamin K for bone health

It is also high in beta-carotene (although its dark green color disguises the orange pigment) and another carotenoid called lutein, which is known to improve visual acuity and to protect against age-related macular degeneration (30).

Spinach also contains zeaxanthin, another antioxidant that protects the eyes from UV damage.

How to eat: Make soup or pasta sauce using frozen chopped spinach. Gently wilt spinach with garlic and olive or coconut oil. Throw a handful in your morning smoothie. Use inside buckwheat wraps or tortillas. Or, just toss in with mixed greens in a salad.

Sprouted Foods

Sprouts have exceptionally concentrated levels of nutrients—first because the seed, grain, or bean they come from contains all the nutrients required to grow a new plant, and because the sprouting process greatly increases the levels of vitamins, minerals, amino acids, essential fatty acids, and enzymes present. The sprouting process releases enzymes that break down some of the nutrients into their constituent parts, making them very bio-available in our bodies.

Sprouted grains are more digestible than ordinary grains and also contain less phytic acid, which can inhibit our absorption of important minerals such as zinc. Sprouting wheat breaks down the gluten so some wheat-intolerant people can eat sprouted wheat bread. Sprouting beans prevents them from releasing gas in the intestinal tract.

Another remarkable property of sprouts is that they contain the nucleic acids RNA and DNA, which are necessary for healthy cell division and thus may protect against cancer. Sprouts are a "living" food and their vitality has a regenerative effect on us when we eat them.

How to eat: Sprouted seeds are available in health food shops. Or, you can easily make them at home in a sprouting jar. Add to salads and stir-fries to make them more filling and nutrient-rich.

Sweet Potatoes

Sweet potatoes are richer in nutrients and lower on the glycemic index than ordinary potatoes. They also have a more succulent flavor.

Sweet potatoes are such an important part of the Okinawan diet that there is even a local greeting, *nmu kamatooin*, meaning, "Are you getting enough sweet potato?" Sweet potatoes contain vitamins E and C, fiber, and minerals, including zinc, copper, magnesium, iron, and phosphorus.

Sweet potatoes also contain more of the antioxidant beta-carotene than any other vegetable—although it is also found in other rich orange-colored foods, such as carrots, pumpkins, and apricots. Your body converts beta-carotene to vitamin A, which helps support the health of the respiratory and digestive tracts. Beta-carotene also accumulates in the skin to protect it against sun damage.

How to eat: Roast, bake, steam, or use in soups and casseroles. Beta-carotene is fat-soluble and will only be absorbed if there is enough fat present, so use salads dressed with olive oil to accompany your sweet potatoes and squash, or roast on a low heat with olive oil or coconut oil.

One oft-cited study of Finnish men showed that giving high doses of beta-carotene in supplement form to smokers increased the risk of lung cancer. However, eating moderate doses as provided by a diet rich in orange and dark green vegetables has been found to have a protective effect against a range of cancers.

Intermittent Blasting Recipes

Tomatoes and Tomato Paste

Tomatoes are the best source of lycopene, the carotenoid responsible for the reds and pinks found in tomatoes, watermelon, rose hips, guavas, and pink grapefruit. Tomatoes and tomato paste are popular in Mediterranean cooking.

Lycopene is best known for its ability to protect against prostate cancer, according to numerous studies (31). One study showed that men with the highest intakes of tomatoes and tomato products had a 35 percent lower risk of prostate cancer and a 53 percent lower risk of aggressive prostate cancer (32).

Tomatoes are also high in vitamin C and folic acid, which probably work in synergy with the lycopene to protect against other illnesses. High blood levels of lycopene are thought to be able to lower heart disease risk in women by up to 50 percent—and one study has shown that lycopene may protect against cervical cancer (33).

Another advantage of eating tomatoes is that they block the formation of carcinogenic compounds called nitrosamines formed when we eat cured meats. So, if you want to eat cured meats, you can limit the damage by having them with a tomato salad.

How to eat: Cook tomatoes with olive oil or coconut oil to improve the absorption of lycopene. Tomato paste, the richest source of lycopene, can be used in casseroles or spread on home-made pizza with garlic, herbs, olives, artichokes, and a moderate amount of cheese. Of course, tomatoes are a delicious addition to a salad.

Turmeric

Bright orange turmeric, a popular spice used in curries and known in India as the spice of life, first stole the spotlight when curry-eating Asians were found to have remarkably low levels of Alzheimer's disease and less cognitive decline.

The magic ingredient in turmeric is curcumin, which:

- Binds to the plaques and tangles which characterize the brains of Alzheimer's patients (34-36).
- Is a powerful anti-inflammatory antioxidant—shown to be as effective as anti-inflammatory drugs, to decrease biomarkers of inflammation, and to improve symptoms of inflammatory bowel disease (37, 38).
- Is a promising treatment for autoimmune diseases like multiple sclerosis, rheumatoid arthritis, psoriasis, thyroiditis, and lupus, thanks to its ability to regulate inflammatory cytokines (39).
- Increases levels of glutathione, an antioxidant that works within cells to protect them from free radical damage and possibly protect against cancer.
- Has a long history of use for liver disorders and might help the liver eliminate cancerous toxins.

Studies also show that curcumin induces apoptosis (cell 'suicide') in cancer cells and inhibits the development of chemically-induced cancers in animals (40, 41).

How to use: Add a teaspoon of turmeric to bean and lentil dishes, casseroles, stews, or marinades for chicken or fish. Mix turmeric into cooked brown rice, or sprinkle on cauliflower. Adding black pepper improves absorption. Juice your favorite fresh organic produce and add turmeric to these juices.

Fermented foods

The friendly bacteria in fermented foods can have a major impact on whether or not our bodies actually absorb the nutrients in our food. We actually have 10 times more bacteria than human cells (10 trillion human cells and 100 trillion bacteria), weighing around 8.8 pounds in total, with up to 1000 different species residing in our GI tract. And their effects on our health cannot be underestimated.

Whether or not we are prone to stomach upsets, the degree to which we metabolize our food, our levels of certain vitamins, our immunity, and other facets of health all depend to a great extent on the bacteria living inside us. Do you eat a modern low-fiber diet? Suffer stress? Have you taken several courses of antibiotics, or do you eat too much sugar? You're likely to have many billion too few friendly bacteria—and far too many unfriendly ones.

Friendly bacteria:

- Synthesize B vitamins and vitamin K
- Produce enzymes to help digest dairy products
- Metabolize phytoestrogens
- Extract calcium from milk
- Aid digestion of protein, glucose, and fiber
- Aid absorption of minerals
- Kill pathogenic bacteria
- Rid the intestinal tract of salmonella, shigella, and e.coli
- Lower cholesterol levels
- Help prevent constipation
- Has anti-tumor effects

Probiotics help maintain the integrity of the digestive tract, thus preventing the excessive intestinal permeability that is linked to food intolerances and allergies.

Superfood References

(1) Langmead L, Feakins RM, Goldthorpe S, et al. Randomized, double-blind, placebo-controlled trial of oral aloe vera gel for active ulcerative colitis. Alimentary pharmacology & therapeutics April 2004;19(7):739-47.

(2) Boudreau MD, Beland FA. An evaluation of the biological and toxicological properties of Aloe barbadensis (miller), Aloe vera. Journal of environmental science and health part C, Environmental carcinogenesis & ecotoxicology reviews April 2006;24(1): 103-54.

(2a) Kametani S, et al. Mechanism of growth inhibitory effect of cape aloe extract in ehrlich ascites tumor cells. J Nutr Sci Vitaminol (Tokyo). 2007 Dec;53(6):540-6.

(2b) Goyal PK, Gehlot P. Radioprotective effects of Aloe vera leaf extract on Swiss albino mice against whole-body gamma irradiation. J Environ Pathol Toxicol Oncol, 2009;28(1):53-61.

(2c) Tamura N, Yoshida T, Miyaji K, Sugita-Konishi Y, Hattori M. Inhibition of infectious diseases by components from Aloe vera. Biosci Biotechnol Biochem. 2009 Apr 23;73(4):950-3. Epub 2009 Apr 7.

(3) Vogler BK, Ernst E. Aloe vera: a systematic review of its clinical effectiveness. Br J Gen Prac 1999;49:823-828.

(4) Schwartz, Steven J. How Can the Metabolomic Response to Lycopene (Exposures, Durations, Intracellular Concentrations) in Humans Be Adequately Evaluated? Journal of Nutrition August 2005;135:2040S-2041S

(5) Lu et al. Inhibition of prostate cancer cell growth by an avocado extract: role of lipid-soluble bioactive substances. J Nutr Biochem, 2005;16(1):23-30.

(6) Shukitt-Hale, B; Lau FC; Joseph JA. Berry Fruit Supplementation and the Aging Brain. Journal of Agricultural and Food Chemistry. 2008;56:636-641.

(7) Verhoeven DT, Verhagen H, Goldbohm RA, van den Brandt PA, van Poppel G. A review of mechanisms underlying anticarcinogenicity by brassica vegetables. Chem Biol Interact. 1997;103(2):79-129. (PubMed).

(8) Conaway CC, Yang YM, Chung FL. Isothiocyanates as cancer chemopreventive agents: their biological activities and metabolism in rodents and humans. Curr Drug Metab. 2002;3(3):233-255. (PubMed).

(9) Fahey JW, Zhang Y, Talalay P. Broccoli sprouts: an exceptionally rich source of inducers of enzymes that protect against chemical carcinogens. Proc Natl Acad Sci USA. 1997;94(19):10367-10372. (PubMed).

(10) Verhoeven DT, Goldbohm RA, van Poppel G, Verhagen H, van den Brandt PA. Epidemiological studies on brassica vegetables and

cancer risk. Cancer Epidemiol Biomarkers Prev. 1996;5(9):733-748. (PubMed).

(11) Raikkonen, Katri; Pesonen, Anu-Katriina; Jarvenpaa, Anna-Liisa; Strandberg, Timo E. Sweet babies: chocolate consumption during pregnancy and infant temperament at 6 months. Early Human Development, 2003; 76 (2); 139-145.

(12) Wu LC, Ho JA, Shieh MC, Lu IW. Antioxidant and Antiproliferative activities of Spirulina and Chlorella water extracts. J Agric Food Chem, 2005 May 18;53(10):4207-12.

(13) Suetsuna K, Chen JR. Identification of antihypertensive peptides from peptic digest of two microalgae, Chlorella vulgaris and Spirulina platensis. Mar Biotechnol (NY). 2001 Jul;3(4):305-9.

(14) Horn-Ross PL, John EM, Canchola AJ, Steward SL, Lee MM. Phytoestrogen intake and endometrial cancer risk. J Natl Cancer Inst. 2003;95(15):1158-1164. (PubMed).

(15) McCann SE, Freudenheim JL, Marshall JR, Graham S. Risk of human ovarian cancer is related to dietary intake of selected nutrients, phytochemicals and food groups. J Nutr. 2003;133(6):1937-1942. (PubMed).

(16) Moruisi KG, Oosthuizen W, Opperman AM. Phytosterols/stanols lower cholesterol concentrations in familial hypercholesterolemic subjects: a systematic review with meta-analysis. J Am Coll Nutr. 2006;25(1):41-48. (PubMed).

(17) Arjmandi BH, Khan DA, Jurna S. Whole flaxseed consumption lowers serum LDL-cholesterol and lipoprotein(a) concentrations in postmenopausal women. Nutr Res. 1998;18:1203-1214.

(18) Awad AB, Fink CS, Williams H, Kim U. In vitro and in vivo (SCID mice) effects of phytosterols on the growth and dissemination of human prostate cancer PC-3 cells. Eur J Cancer Prev. 2001;10(6):507-513. (PubMed).

(19) Awad AB, Downie A, Fink CS, Kim U. Dietary phytosterol inhibits the growth and metastasis of MDA-MB-231 human breast cancer cells grown in SCID mice. Anticancer Res. 2000;20(2A):821-824 (PubMed).

(20) De Stefani E, Boffetta P, Ronco AL, et al. Plant sterols and risk of stomach cancer: a case-control study in Uruguay. Nutr Cancer. 2000;37(2):140-144. (PubMed).

(21) Mendilaharsu M, De Stefani E, Deneo-Pellegrini H, Carzoglio J, Ronco A. Phytosterols and risk of lung cancer: a case-control study in Uruguay. Lung Cancer. 1998;21(1):37-45.

(22) Fleischauer AT, Poole C, Arab L. Garlic consumption and cancer prevention: meta-analyses of colorectal and stomach cancers. Am J Clin Nutr. 2000; 72(4):1047-1052. (PubMed).

(23) Song K, Milner JA. Heating garlic inhibits its ability to suppress 7, 12-dimethylbenz(a)anthracene-induced DNA adduct formation in rat mammary tissue. J Nutr. 1999;129(3):657-661. (PubMed).

(24) Nigam N, George J, Srivastava S, Roy P, Bhui K, Singh M, Shukla Y. Induction of apoptosis by [6]-gingerol associated with the modulation of p53 and involvement of mitochondrial signaling pathway in B[a]P-induced mouse skin tumorigenesis. Cancer Chemother Pharmacol. 2009 Jul 24.

(25) Rao BN, Rao BS, Aithal BK, Kumar MR. Radiomodifying and anticlastogenic effect of zingerone on Swiss albino mice exposed to whole body gamma radiation. Mutat Res. 2009 Jun-Jul;677(1-2):33-41. (PubMed).

(26) Oguni I, Cheng ShuJun, Annual Report of the Skylark Food Science Institute, no. 3.57(1991).

(27) Ahmad, N. et al. Green Tea Constituent epigallocatechin-3-gallate and Induction of Apoptosis and Cell Cycle Arrest in Human Carcinoma Cells. Journal of the National Cancer Institute 89, no 24 (1997):1881-1886.

(28) Kodama N, Komuta K, Sakai N, & Nanba H. Effects of D-fraction, a polysaccharide from Grifola frondosa on Tumor Growth Involve Activation of NK Cells. Biological & Pharmaceutical Bulletin 25, no. 12 (December 2002): 1647-1650.

(29) Peeters PH, Keinan-Boker L, van der Schouw YT, Grobbee DE. Phytoestrogens and breast cancer risk. Review of the epidemiological evidence. Breast Cancer Res Treat. 2003;77(2):171-183. (PubMed).

(30) Mares-Perlman JA, Millen AE, Ficek TL, Hankinson SE. The body of evidence to support a protective role for lutein and zeaxanthin in delaying chronic disease. Overview. J. Nutr. 2002;132(3):518S-524S. (PubMed).

(31) Giovannucci E. A review of epidemiologic studies of tomatoes, lycopene and prostate cancer. Exp Biol Med (Maywood). 2002;227(10):852-859. (PubMed).

(32) Giovannucci E, Ascherio A, Rimm EB, Stampfer MJ, Colditz GA, Willet WC. Intake of carotenoids and retinol in relation to risk of prostate cancer. J Natl Cancer Inst. 1995;87(23):1767-1776. (PubMed).

(33) Van Eenwyk, J; Davis, FG, Bowne, PE. Dietary and Serum Carotenoids and Cervical Intraepithelial Neoplasia. International Journal of Cancer 48 (1991):34-38.

(34) Yang F, Lim GP, Begum AN, et al. Curcumin inhibits formation of amyloid beta oligomers and fibrils, binds plaques, and reduces amyloid in vivo. J Biol Chem. 2005;280(7):5892-5901. (PubMed).

(35) Lim GP, Chu T, Yang F, Beech W, Frautschy SA, Cole GM. The curry spice curcumin reduces oxidative damage and amyloid pathology in an Alzheimer transgenic mouse. J Neurosci. 2001;21(21):8370-8377. (PubMed).

(36) Frautschy SA, Hu W, Kim P, et al. Phenolic anti-inflammatory antioxidant reversal of Abeta-induced cognitive deficits and neuropathology. Neurobiol Agin. 2001;22(6):993-1005. (PubMed).

(37) Deodhar SD, Sethi R, Srimal RC. Preliminary study on antirheumatic activity of curcumin (diferuloylmethane). Indian J Med Res, 1980;71:632-634.

(38) Hanai H, Sugimoto K. Curcumin has bright prospects for the treatment of inflammatory bowel disease. Curr Pharm Des. 2009;15(18):2087-94. (PubMed).

(39) Bright, JJ. Curcumin and autoimmune disease. Adv Exp Med Biol. 2007;595:425-51. (PubMed).

(40) Sharma RA, Gescher AJ, Steward WP. Curcumin: The story so far. Eur J Cancer. 2005;41(13):1955-1968. (PubMed).

(41) Huang MT, Lou YR, Ma W, Newmark HL, Reuhl KR, Conney AH. Inhibitory effects of dietary curcumin on forestomach,

duodenal, and colon carcinogenesis in mice. *Cancer Research.* 1994;54(22):5841-5847. (PubMed).

Chapter 7: Healthy Life Overview

ABB - "Always Be Blasting"

There's a strategy in sales abbreviated as ABC, which stands for "Always Be Closing." Considering 95 percent of Americans are deficient in nutrition and we are experiencing epidemic rates of chronic disease, I believe we should adopt a strategy of ABB; "Always Be Blasting." We need to blast our bodies with high-quality nutrition at every opportunity. Anytime we eat, we have a choice of what we put into our bodies: a choice of putting in junk food with little or no nutritional value, or consuming superfoods and blasting our bodies with quality nutrients. Keeping this in mind will help you consume the very best nutrition available every time you eat, whether you are on a Blast or not.

Living a Healthy Life

Intermittent Blasting is a great tool for managing weight and restoring health. As we have discussed throughout this book, our health in the modern world is suffering. We as a people are suffering. Chronic disease is rampant and has become an expected and accepted part of life. Intermittent Blasting is a way people living in a modern society can lose weight and improve their health. But overall, we need to rethink our lifestyle from a larger perspective. One that combines science, modernization and food processing in healthier ways, not just profitable and convenient ones. Because when we, as a society, are unhealthy we all suffer, both health-wise and economically.

A Healthy Diet in a Nutshell

Food Groups to Include:

- Vegetables and salads: At least three servings of vegetables at lunch and three at supper—including garlic and onions and

dark green leafy vegetables (e.g., broccoli, spinach, bell peppers, zucchini, lettuce, carrots, cucumber, celery, celeriac, fennel, sweet potatoes, green beans, green peas, etc.).
- Fruits: Daily - One to three pieces.
- Grains: If you choose to include grains, choose whole grains in moderate quantities instead of refined grains. These include oats, millet, rye, barley, brown rice, red rice, quinoa, buckwheat, amaranth, and whole wheat.
- Vegetable proteins: Daily or most days - nuts, beans, lentils, miso, seeds, flax seeds, chia seeds, and sprouted seeds.
- Animal proteins: In moderate to small quantities - eggs from cage free-chickens, fish from an unpolluted source, live plain yogurt, lean organic beef, organic cheese from goat's or sheep's milk, lean organic poultry.
- Monounsaturated fats: Daily or most days - from unheated extra virgin olive oil, avocados, seeds, nuts; if cooking with olive oil, keep the heat low and cooking time short.
- Omega 3 essential fatty acids: Daily - oily fish, ground or soaked flax seed, chia seed, walnuts, nutritional supplements.
- Omega 6 essential fatty acids: Daily - nuts and seeds, avocado, some oils, ground flax seed, chia seed.
- Fermented foods: Small amounts daily, or several times per week - traditionally marinated vegetables, sauerkraut, miso, tempeh, olives, live plain yogurt, kefir, and kefir water.
- Water: Several glasses daily, sipped throughout the day. At least 1/2 ounce per pound of bodyweight.
- Green tea, herb tea: Daily as desired.
- Red wine: Stick to small amounts of organic red wine, with a meal. If you drink alcohol, red wine has the most health advantages and the fewest disadvantages.
- Fiber: Daily, both soluble and insoluble, sourced in your fruits, vegetables, nuts, seeds, and grains.

Food Groups to Restrict/Exclude:

- Refined sugar
- Refined carbs (white flour, white rice)
- Alcohol
- Caffeine
- Trans fats from processed foods
- Damaged fats from cooking oils
- Non-organic dairy products

Cooking Tips

- Use fresh, local, organic produce when possible.
- Use meat as a flavoring for a dish, rather than making it the "star" of the meal.
- Use organic pasture-raised, grass-fed meat when possible.
- Use herbs and spices to flavor recipes, rather than lots of refined salt. Experiment with some that you haven't used before—the internet is a great resource for finding out how to use new herbs & spices. Use Celtic Sea Salt, Himalayan Pink or Real Salt when using salt.
- Use filtered water when a recipe calls for water.
- Boiling or poaching is best to preserve the nutrients in eggs; second-best is scrambled.
- Remember not to overcook vegetables. Lightly steaming, gently roasting, or just eating raw are preferred methods.
- Toss together different colors of vegetables to arouse your eyes and taste buds.
- Use first cold-pressed olive oil in salads and when drizzling over other foods.
- Use coconut oil when cooking at higher heat.
- Steam or slow-roast vegetables. Or eat them raw to preserve vitamins, minerals, and enzymes.
- Avoid burning or charring meat. This can create pro-aging free radicals and carcinogenic heterocyclic aromatic amines (HAAs). Grill with indirect heat only.

Intermittent Blasting Recipes

- Use fresh herbs, garlic, lemon, and spices such as turmeric liberally in your food preparation for flavor.
- Try to consume foods grown and prepared locally to ensure they are as fresh as possible.
- Avoid frying. It damages oils and can make them unhealthy.
- If pan-searing or frying, use oils with a very high smoke point, such as coconut (preferred), red palm or avocado oils. These oils are more stable at higher temperatures than corn or olive oil.
- Use meat and dairy products as a condiment to flavor vegetable dishes, rather than using them as the main feature of your dishes.

Shopping Tips

- Read labels.
- When grocery shopping, choose locally- grown produce and meats - no chemicals, processing, or preservatives.
- Keep to the perimeter of the grocery store, where the fresh produce tends to be. Avoid the interior aisles, where the chips and other junk foods tend to be.
- On the interior aisles, avoid the UFOs - unidentified food objects. You'll know them when you see ingredients that are artificial, unrecognizable and unpronounceable.
- When purchasing fruits and vegetables, always look for labels such as Local, Organic, and No GMO (genetically modified organisms).
- If you can't find fresh produce, your second choice should be frozen fruits and vegetables. Canned foods are lower in nutrients.
- Look for free-range, organic beef and poultry products. Levels of harmful chemicals should be much lower than in the products of industrial-farmed animals.
- Choose deep-water, wild-caught ocean fish, which is likely to have lower levels of mercury, PCBs, dioxin, and other toxic,

cancer-causing chemicals. Avoid farm-raised fish. Wild-caught Alaskan salmon is preferred.
- Avoid having tuna more than twice per month. It can be high in mercury. Choose tuna caught by the pole-and-line method.
- When buying breads, choose one hundred percent whole grain rather than white breads made with refined flours. Avoid high-calorie pastries altogether.
- Avoid high-sugar snacks. Choose whole-grain crackers or baked snacks.
- Try to buy nuts in their shells, since the oils in pre-shelled nuts go rancid quickly. Children love cracking the shells open, so it's a great way to eat nuts.
- Choose water, fresh juice, herbal tea, and organic, fair-trade coffee over sugary soft drinks and avoid diet soft drinks and other diet beverages that contain harmful chemicals
- "Sugar-free" on the label only refers to sucrose or table sugar. Other sugars to watch for are fructose, maltose, lactose, glucose, dextrose, corn-syrup solids, corn sweeteners, and hydrolyzed corn starch.
- Look for products with healthier sweeteners, such as fruit, stevia, evaporated cane juice, or agave. Try sweetening your coffee and tea with raw honey instead of table sugar.
- Use Celtic Sea Salt, Himalayan Pink salt or Real Salt brand salt rather than refined table salt, as they are unrefined and contain beneficial minerals.
- When buying soaps, lotions, cleaners, and detergents, look for unscented products. Items with fragrances may contain potentially harmful chemicals.
- Avoid antibacterial soaps with the chemicals triclosan and triclocarban. They're thought to affect reproductive hormones as well as the nervous system and might contribute to the evolution of antibiotic-resistant superbugs.

Become a Locavore

Always choose fresh local foods when possible. Most produce travels an average of 2000 miles before it reaches our table, which presents several problems. First, nutrients begin to degrade once the food is harvested, and ideally you want as much nutrition as possible. Second, produce that travels long distances must be harvested well before it reaches maturity, which means less time for the food to absorb minerals and synthesize vitamins from the soil. Buying locally, you'll enjoy fresher, tastier, and healthier food, while also supporting small, local farmers in your community and leaving a much lower carbon footprint.

Buy Organic When Possible

Today when we purchase organic food, it seems as though we are purchasing something special, something a little more gourmet. What we have to hunt for and make special requests for, what we call organic food, our grandparents simply referred to as food. If you think about it, we really shouldn't have to make special requests and go out of our way to buy food free of poisons. Alas, this is the current situation as a result of industrialized food production and we have to deal with it as best we can.

Non-organic foods have been shown to contain chemicals such as pesticides, herbicides, fungicides, which have been shown to damage health and even cause neurological disorders. They also contain less nutrition. So buy organic when possible and be sure to wash thoroughly when using conventionally grown foods.

Foods most likely to contain chemical (pesticides, herbicides, fungicides) residue:

- Apples
- Bell peppers
- Beets

Intermittent Blasting Recipes

- Blueberries
- Broccoli
- Butter
- Carrots
- Celery
- Cherries
- Citrus (if using for zest)
- Corn (sweet, frozen)
- Cucumbers
- Dairy (milk, yogurt, cottage cheese, cream cheese, ice cream, etc.)
- Fatty meats (grass-fed, if possible)
- Grapes (both domestic & imported)
- Green beans
- Green onions
- Greens (kale, collards, Swiss chard, etc.)
- Hot peppers
- Lettuce
- Nectarines
- Peaches
- Pears
- Potatoes (white, red, gold)
- Radishes
- Raspberries
- Snow & sugar snap peas
- Spinach
- Strawberries
- Summer squash (zucchini, yellow squash, crookneck, pattypan, etc.)
- Tomatoes (cherry)
- Turnips
- Yogurt

Least likely to contain chemical residue:

Intermittent Blasting Recipes

- Asparagus
- Avocados
- Bananas
- Cabbage
- Cauliflower
- Citrus (if eating inside only)
- Corn, sweet, fresh (non-GMO only)
- Eggplants
- Kiwis
- Mangoes
- Melons (cantaloupe, honeydew, watermelon)
- Onions, dry bulb (any color)
- Papayas
- Peas (sweet, frozen)
- Pineapples
- Shallots
- Sweet potatoes

How to Prepare Vegetables

Oven-Roasted Vegetables

Roughly chop vegetables suitable for roasting, such as squash, pumpkin, sweet potato, potato, leeks, fennel, carrots, onion, and garlic. Drizzle with coconut oil or olive oil, season, and roast on a low heat, stirring occasionally, until done. Towards the end of roasting add herbs, such as rosemary or thyme. Salt and pepper to taste.

Stir-fried vegetables

Slice vegetables suitable for stir-frying, such as carrots, snow peas, green beans, bell peppers, broccoli, cauliflower, onion, and garlic. Stir-fry on medium to low heat (if the oil smokes, it's too hot) with coconut oil, red palm oil, or olive oil (at lower temperature) and soy sauce, or steam-fry in stock. Cook for a short time so that the vegetables still have a bit of crunch to them.

Steamed vegetables

Steaming vegetables for a short time is a very healthy way to cook them. Steaming is better than boiling, since boiling causes minerals to leach into the cooking water, and steaming is also quick and easy. Sweet potatoes, broccoli, snow peas, green beans, asparagus, squash, carrots, and most green vegetables are great for steaming. Serve with a drizzle of olive oil or butter, garlic, lemon, and any seasoning you prefer. You can steam vegetables in water or stock.

Beans and Lentils

When using beans or lentils, you can either use canned legumes or dried legumes that have been soaked overnight and cooked. The latter is preferable health-wise since dried, cooked legumes are of higher quality than canned, but canned beans are certainly quicker and easier. Therefore, use canned beans if necessary, but try to buy good-quality organic varieties.

Choose only organic animal products

Meat and dairy products from animals raised on an organic diet free of growth-hormones and antibiotics are living a natural life outdoors are much healthier than mass-produced animals raised on a factory farm (mass produced meats are found in most U.S. groceries).

Factory-farmed animals eat foods that are foreign to their natural diet—like soy and corn and most of it is genetically modified. These types of feed make the animals grow very quickly, but it also makes their flesh and dairy products unnaturally low in omega 3 fatty acids. Moreover, you are actually consuming harmful chemicals (once consumed by the animal) when you eat these types of products.

On the other hand, pasture-fed, free-range, and wild game fed grass and other natural wild plant foods are much healthier and higher in nutrients. Their native diet makes their flesh much higher in beneficial monounsaturated and polyunsaturated fats.

Made in United States
Orlando, FL
17 May 2022